Outcomes and Therapeutic Management of Bladder Cancer

Outcomes and Therapeutic Management of Bladder Cancer

Editor

Marco Moschini

MDPI • Basel • Beijing • Wuhan • Barcelona • Belgrade • Manchester • Tokyo • Cluj • Tianjin

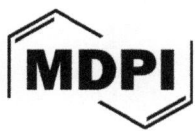

Editor
Marco Moschini
Univ Vita Salute San Raffaele
Italy

Editorial Office
MDPI
St. Alban-Anlage 66
4052 Basel, Switzerland

This is a reprint of articles from the Special Issue published online in the open access journal *Journal of Clinical Medicine* (ISSN 2077-0383) (available at: https://www.mdpi.com/journal/jcm/special_issues/Outcomes_TherapManag_BC).

For citation purposes, cite each article independently as indicated on the article page online and as indicated below:

LastName, A.A.; LastName, B.B.; LastName, C.C. Article Title. *Journal Name* **Year**, *Article Number*, Page Range.

ISBN 978-3-03936-934-8 (Hbk)
ISBN 978-3-03936-935-5 (PDF)

© 2020 by the authors. Articles in this book are Open Access and distributed under the Creative Commons Attribution (CC BY) license, which allows users to download, copy and build upon published articles, as long as the author and publisher are properly credited, which ensures maximum dissemination and a wider impact of our publications.

The book as a whole is distributed by MDPI under the terms and conditions of the Creative Commons license CC BY-NC-ND.

Contents

About the Editor vii

Marco Moschini
From Basic Science to Clinical Research to Develop New Solutions to Improve Diagnoses and Treatment of Bladder Cancer Patients
Reprinted from: *J. Clin. Med.* **2020**, *9*, 2373, doi:10.3390/jcm9082373 1

Guillaume Ploussard, Benjamin Pradere, Jean-Baptiste Beauval, Christine Chevreau, Christophe Almeras, Etienne Suc, Jean-Romain Gautier, Anne-Pascale Laurenty, Mathieu Roumiguié, Guillaume Loison, Christophe Tollon, Loïc Mourey, Ambroise Salin, Evanguelos Xylinas and Damien Pouessel
Survival Outcomes of Patients with Pathologically Proven Positive Lymph Nodes at Time of Radical Cystectomy with or without Neoadjuvant Chemotherapy
Reprinted from: *J. Clin. Med.* **2020**, *9*, 1962, doi:10.3390/jcm9061962 5

Donghyun Kim, Jin Man Kim, Jun-Sang Kim, Sup Kim and Kyung-Hee Kim
Differential Expression and Clinicopathological Significance of HER2, Indoleamine 2,3-Dioxygenase and PD-L1 in Urothelial Carcinoma of the Bladder
Reprinted from: *J. Clin. Med.* **2020**, *9*, 1265, doi:10.3390/jcm9051265 15

Danijel Sikic, Markus Eckstein, Ralph M. Wirtz, Jonas Jarczyk, Thomas S. Worst, Stefan Porubsky, Bastian Keck, Frank Kunath, Veronika Weyerer, Johannes Breyer, Wolfgang Otto, Sebastien Rinaldetti, Christian Bolenz, Arndt Hartmann, Bernd Wullich and Philipp Erben
FOXA1 Gene Expression for Defining Molecular Subtypes of Muscle-Invasive Bladder Cancer after Radical Cystectomy
Reprinted from: *J. Clin. Med.* **2020**, *9*, 994, doi:10.3390/jcm9040994 31

Sara Monteiro-Reis, Ana Blanca, Joana Tedim-Moreira, Isa Carneiro, Diana Montezuma, Paula Monteiro, Jorge Oliveira, Luís Antunes, Rui Henrique, António Lopez-Beltran and Carmen Jerónimo
A Multiplex Test Assessing $MiR663a_{me}$ and VIM_{me} in Urine Accurately Discriminates Bladder Cancer from Inflammatory Conditions
Reprinted from: *J. Clin. Med.* **2020**, *9*, 605, doi:10.3390/jcm9020605 45

Gabriele Tuderti, Riccardo Mastroianni, Simone Flammia, Mariaconsiglia Ferriero, Costantino Leonardo, Umberto Anceschi, Aldo Brassetti, Salvatore Guaglianone, Michele Gallucci and Giuseppe Simone
Sex-Sparing Robot-Assisted Radical Cystectomy with Intracorporeal Padua Ileal Neobladder in Female: Surgical Technique, Perioperative, Oncologic and Functional Outcomes
Reprinted from: *J. Clin. Med.* **2020**, *9*, 577, doi:10.3390/jcm9020577 57

Zhengqiu Zhou, Connor J. Kinslow, Peng Wang, Bin Huang, Simon K. Cheng, Israel Deutsch, Matthew S. Gentry and Ramon C. Sun
Clear Cell Adenocarcinoma of the Urinary Bladder Is a Glycogen-Rich Tumor with Poorer Prognosis
Reprinted from: *J. Clin. Med.* **2020**, *9*, 138, doi:10.3390/jcm9010138 67

Claudia Claroni, Marco Covotta, Giulia Torregiani, Maria Elena Marcelli, Gabriele Tuderti, Giuseppe Simone, Alessandra Scotto di Uccio, Antonio Zinilli and Ester Forastiere
Recovery from Anesthesia after Robotic-Assisted Radical Cystectomy: Two Different Reversals of Neuromuscular Blockade
Reprinted from: *J. Clin. Med.* **2019**, *8*, 1774, doi:10.3390/jcm8111774 . . . . **79**

Florian Janisch, Hang Yu, Malte W. Vetterlein, Roland Dahlem, Oliver Engel, Margit Fisch, Shahrokh F. Shariat, Armin Soave and Michael Rink
Do Younger Patients with Muscle-Invasive Bladder Cancer have Better Outcomes?
Reprinted from: *J. Clin. Med.* **2019**, *8*, 1459, doi:10.3390/jcm8091459 . . . . **89**

Marco Moschini, Stefania Zamboni, Francesco Soria, Romain Mathieu, Evanguelos Xylinas, Wei Shen Tan, John D Kelly, Giuseppe Simone, Anoop Meraney, Suprita Krishna, Badrinath Konety, Agostino Mattei, Philipp Baumeister, Livio Mordasini, Francesco Montorsi, Alberto Briganti, Andrea Gallina, Armando Stabile, Rafael Sanchez-Salas, Xavier Cathelineau, Michael Rink, Andrea Necchi, Pierre I. Karakiewicz, Morgan Rouprêt, Anthony Koupparis, Wassim Kassouf, Douglas S Scherr, Guillaume Ploussard, Stephen A. Boorjian, Yair Lotan, Prasanna Sooriakumaran and Shahrokh F. Shariat
Open Versus Robotic Cystectomy: A Propensity Score Matched Analysis Comparing Survival Outcomes
Reprinted from: *J. Clin. Med.* **2019**, *8*, 1192, doi:10.3390/jcm8081192 . . . . **99**

About the Editor

Marco Moschini completed his medical degree in 2012, at Vita Salute-San Raffaele University—Milan, followed by his PhD in 2016, at Universita Magna Graecia. He embarked upon a one-year fellowship at the Department of Urology of the Mayo Clinic in Rochester in 2015, and a one-year fellowship at the Department of Urology of the General Hospital of Vienna. He spent one year as a surgical robotic fellow in Paris (Institute Mutualiste Montsouris). He has currently in residency in Urology in Luzern (Switzerland), and has been since 2017. Since 2017, Moschini has been an active member of the EAU's Young Academic Urologists' Urothelial Cancer Group. He is an associate editor of *Swiss Urology*, and has been the guest associate editor of an edition of *Translational Andrology and Urology (TAU)*, based on non-muscle invasive bladder cancer, and for an edition of *Arab Journal of Urology*, on the same topic. He is the author of more than 200 peer-reviewed articles in international journals; more than 50 as first author. He serves as reviewer for more than 30 urological and oncological journals. His main interest regards urologic oncology, with a focus on bladder, upper urinary tract and prostate cancers. He is the associated editor for the educational platform of the EAU on urothelial cancer.

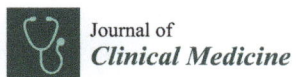

Editorial

From Basic Science to Clinical Research to Develop New Solutions to Improve Diagnoses and Treatment of Bladder Cancer Patients

Marco Moschini [1,2]

1. Department of Urology, San Raffaele Scientific Institute, Urological Research Institute, 20132 Milan, Italy; marco.moschini87@gmail.com
2. Luzerner Kantonsspital, Spitalstrasse, CH-6000 Luzern, Switzerland

Received: 20 July 2020; Accepted: 21 July 2020; Published: 25 July 2020

Bladder cancer (BCa) is the tenth most common form of cancer worldwide, with 549,000 new cases and 200,000 deaths estimated in 2018 [1]. To address the several unmet questions in the field of BCa research, recently the European Association of Urology (EAU) and the European Society of Medical Oncology (ESMO) selected a panel of experts to define important topics in the field of BCa and to propose possible management solutions [2,3]. In this Special Issue on outcomes and therapeutic management of bladder cancer, we collected a series of articles treating some of the most important topics for the urological community. First, the use of robotic surgery in the treatment of BCa is rapidly increasing, surpassing the use of open surgery in tertiary referral centers [4]. In this regard, literature reporting the efficacy of this technique, in comparison to the old standard, is rapidly increasing [5]. In this issue, we found in a big multicenter collaboration the equivalence of open versus robotic radical cystectomy (RC) in the treatment of BCa patients [6]. Second, functional outcomes after radical cystectomy need to be further reported and investigated to increase the quality of life of BCa patients. Tuderti et al. [7] reported their experience of patients treated with sex sparing robot-assisted radical cystectomy in female patients receiving an intracorporeal neobladder reporting good oncological and functional outcomes 12 months after treatment. From the same institution, Claroni et al. [8] reported on recovery outcomes from anesthesia after robotic-assisted RC.

Third, basic science needs to increase the outcome classification of BCa and the efficacy of diagnostic strategies for an early diagnosis in patients with their first episode of BCa and promptly diagnose a recurrence of BCa in patients who have been already treated. Kim et al. [9] and Sikic et al. [10] and Montero-Reis et al. [11] proposed with different techniques potential markers and therapeutic targets that could improve clinical practices in the future. Fourth, the careful evaluation of variant histology can impact survival outcomes and similarly define optimal treatment strategies by proposing different diagnostic and therapeutic approaches in those patients affected by non-urothelial BCa tumors [12]. Zhou et al. [13] reported on survival outcomes of patients affected by clear cell adenocarcinoma, finding poorer prognosis compared to urothelial cancer. These results confirmed previous findings on this topic [14]. Finally, in this regard the impact of local surgery on patients affected by metastatic BCa is one of the new studied areas in this field [15,16]. I would like to thank the editorial office, authors, reviewers and all the readers for their efforts in putting together this series.

References

1. Bray, F.; Ferlay, J.; Soerjomataram, I.; Siegel, R.L.; Torre, L.A.; Jemal, A. Global cancer statistics 2018: GLOBOCAN estimates of incidence and mortality worldwide for 36 cancers in 185 countries. *CA Cancer J. Clin.* **2018**, *68*, 394–424. [CrossRef]
2. Witjes, J.A.; Babjuk, M.; Bellmunt, J.; Bruins, H.M.; De Reijke, T.M.; De Santis, M.; Gillessen, S.; James, N.; MacLennan, S.; Palou, J.; et al. EAU-ESMO Consensus Statements on the Management of Advanced and Variant Bladder Cancer—An International Collaborative Multistakeholder Effort†. *Eur. Urol.* **2020**, *77*, 223–250. [CrossRef]
3. Horwich, A.; Babjuk, M.; Bellmunt, J.; Bruins, H.; De Reijke, T.; De Santis, M.; Gillessen, S.; James, N.; MacLennan, S.; Palou, J.; et al. EAU–ESMO consensus statements on the management of advanced and variant bladder cancer—An international collaborative multi-stakeholder effort: Under the auspices of the EAU and ESMO Guidelines Committees. *Ann. Oncol.* **2019**, *30*, 1697–1727. [CrossRef]
4. Zamboni, S.; Shariat, S.F.; Mathieu, R.; Xylinas, E.; Abufaraj, M.; D'Andrea, D.; Tan, W.S.; Kelly, J.D.; Simone, G.; Gallucci, M.; et al. Differences in trends in the use of robot-assisted and open radical cystectomy and changes over time in peri-operative outcomes among selected centres in North America and Europe: An international multicentre collaboration. *BJU Int.* **2019**, *124*, 656–664. [CrossRef]
5. Shariat, S.F.; Moschini, M.; D'Andrea, D.; Abufaraj, M.; Foerster, B.; Mathieu, R.; Gust, K.M.; Gontero, P.; Simone, G.; Meraney, A.; et al. Comparative Effectiveness in Perioperative Outcomes of Robotic versus Open Radical Cystectomy: Results from a Multicenter Contemporary Retrospective Cohort Study. *Eur. Urol. Focus* **2018**. [CrossRef]
6. Moschini, M.; Zamboni, S.; Shariat, S.F.; Mathieu, R.; Xylinas, E.; Tan, W.S.; Kelly, J.D.; Simone, G.; Meraney, A.; Krishna, S.; et al. Open Versus Robotic Cystectomy: A Propensity Score Matched Analysis Comparing Survival Outcomes. *J. Clin. Med.* **2019**, *8*, 1192. [CrossRef]
7. Tuderti, G.; Mastroianni, R.; Flammia, S.; Ferriero, M.; Leonardo, C.; Anceschi, U.; Brassetti, A.; Guaglianone, S.; Gallucci, M.; Simone, G. Sex-Sparing Robot-Assisted Radical Cystectomy with Intracorporeal Padua Ileal Neobladder in Female: Surgical Technique, Perioperative, Oncologic and Functional Outcomes. *J. Clin. Med.* **2020**, *9*, 577. [CrossRef]
8. Claroni, C.; Covotta, M.; Torregiani, G.; Marcelli, M.E.; Tuderti, G.; Simone, G.; Di Uccio, A.S.; Zinilli, A.; Forastiere, E. Recovery from Anesthesia after Robotic-Assisted Radical Cystectomy: Two Different Reversals of Neuromuscular Blockade. *J. Clin. Med.* **2019**, *8*, 1774. [CrossRef]
9. Kim, D.; Kim, J.M.; Kim, J.-S.; Kim, S.; Kim, K.-H. Differential Expression and Clinicopathological Significance of HER2, Indoleamine 2,3-Dioxygenase and PD-L1 in Urothelial Carcinoma of the Bladder. *J. Clin. Med.* **2020**, *9*, 1265. [CrossRef]
10. Sikic, D.; Eckstein, M.; Wirtz, R.; Jarczyk, J.; Worst, T.S.; Porubsky, S.; Keck, B.; Kunath, F.; Weyerer, V.; Breyer, J.; et al. FOXA1 Gene Expression for Defining Molecular Subtypes of Muscle-Invasive Bladder Cancer after Radical Cystectomy. *J. Clin. Med.* **2020**, *9*, 994. [CrossRef] [PubMed]
11. Monteiro-Reis, S.; Blanca, A.; Tedim-Moreira, J.; Carneiro, I.; Felizardo, D.; Monteiro, P.; Oliveira, J.; Antunes, L.; Henrique, R.; Lopez-Beltran, A.; et al. A Multiplex Test Assessing MiR663ame and VIMme in Urine Accurately Discriminates Bladder Cancer from Inflammatory Conditions. *J. Clin. Med.* **2020**, *9*, 605. [CrossRef] [PubMed]
12. Abufaraj, M.; Foerster, B.; Schernhammer, E.; Moschini, M.; Kimura, S.; Hassler, M.R.; Preston, M.A.; Karakiewicz, P.I.; Remzi, M.; Shariat, S.F. Micropapillary Urothelial Carcinoma of the Bladder: A Systematic Review and Meta-analysis of Disease Characteristics and Treatment Outcomes. *Eur. Urol.* **2018**, *75*, 649–658. [CrossRef] [PubMed]
13. Zhou, Z.; Kinslow, C.J.; Wang, P.; Huang, B.; Cheng, S.K.; Deutsch, I.; Gentry, M.S.; Sun, R.C. Clear Cell Adenocarcinoma of the Urinary Bladder Is a Glycogen-Rich Tumor with Poorer Prognosis. *J. Clin. Med.* **2020**, *9*, 138. [CrossRef] [PubMed]
14. Moschini, M.; D'Andrea, D.; Korn, S.; Irmak, Y.; Shariat, S.F.; Compérat, E.; Shariat, S.F. Characteristics and clinical significance of histological variants of bladder cancer. *Nat. Rev. Urol.* **2017**, *14*, 651–668. [CrossRef] [PubMed]

15. Abufaraj, M.; Gust, K.; Moschini, M.; Foerster, B.; Soria, F.; Mathieu, R.; Shariat, S.F. Management of muscle invasive, locally advanced and metastatic urothelial carcinoma of the bladder: A literature review with emphasis on the role of surgery. *Transl. Androl. Urol.* **2016**, *5*, 735–744. [CrossRef] [PubMed]
16. Moschini, M.; Xylinas, E.; Zamboni, S.; Mattei, A.; Niegisch, G.; Yu, E.Y.; Bamias, A.; Agarwal, N.; Sridhar, S.S.; Sternberg, C.N.; et al. Efficacy of Surgery in the Primary Tumor Site for Metastatic Urothelial Cancer: Analysis of an International, Multicenter, Multidisciplinary Database. *Eur. Urol. Oncol.* **2020**, *3*, 94–101. [CrossRef] [PubMed]

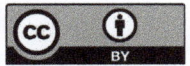

© 2020 by the author. Licensee MDPI, Basel, Switzerland. This article is an open access article distributed under the terms and conditions of the Creative Commons Attribution (CC BY) license (http://creativecommons.org/licenses/by/4.0/).

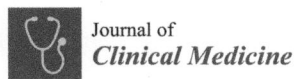

Article

Survival Outcomes of Patients with Pathologically Proven Positive Lymph Nodes at Time of Radical Cystectomy with or without Neoadjuvant Chemotherapy

Guillaume Ploussard [1,*], Benjamin Pradere [2,3], Jean-Baptiste Beauval [1], Christine Chevreau [4], Christophe Almeras [1], Etienne Suc [5], Jean-Romain Gautier [1], Anne-Pascale Laurenty [5], Mathieu Roumiguié [6], Guillaume Loison [1], Christophe Tollon [1], Loïc Mourey [4], Ambroise Salin [1], Evanguelos Xylinas [7] and Damien Pouessel [4]

[1] Department of Urology, La Croix du Sud Hospital, 31130 Quint Fonsegrives, France; jbbeauval@gmail.com (J.-B.B.); c.almeras@gmail.com (C.A.); gautierjr@hotmail.fr (J.-R.G.); guillaumeloison@gmail.com (G.L.); tol@club-internet.fr (C.T.); ambroise.salin@gmail.com (A.S.)
[2] Department of Urology, Bretonneau Hospital, 37000 Tours, France; benjaminpradere@gmail.com
[3] Department of Urology, Comprehensive Cancer Center, Medical University of Vienna, 1090 Vienna, Austria
[4] Department of Oncology, IUCT-O, 31000 Toulouse, France; chevreau.christine@iuct-oncopole.fr (C.C.); mourey.loic@iuct-oncopole.fr (L.M.); pouessel.damien@iuct-oncopole.fr (D.P.)
[5] Department of Oncology, La Croix du Sud Hospital, 31130 Quint Fonsegrives, France; esucsjl@club-internet.fr (E.S.); aplaurenty@capio.fr (A.-P.L.)
[6] Department of Urology, CHU-IUC, 31000 Toulouse, France; roumiguie_mathieu@yahoo.fr
[7] Department of Urology, Bichat-Claude Bernard Hospital, Assistance Publique-Hopitaux de Paris, Paris University, 75018 Paris, France; evanguelosxylinas@hotmail.com
* Correspondence: g.ploussard@gmail.com

Received: 26 May 2020; Accepted: 22 June 2020; Published: 23 June 2020

Abstract: Background: To compare overall survival (OS) outcomes in pN1-3 disease at the time of radical cystectomy (RC) for muscle invasive bladder according to the neoadjuvant chemotherapy (NAC) status. Materials and Methods: This multicenter study included 450 consecutive patients undergoing RC for muscle-invasive urothelial bladder cancer with pN1-3 pM0 disease from 2010 to 2019. NAC consisted in platinum-based chemotherapy. The primary endpoint was the comparison between NAC and non-NAC in terms of death from any cause. OS was assessed using the Kaplan–Meier method and multivariate Cox proportional hazards regression was used to estimate adjusted hazard ratios. Results: Median age was 69 years. Patients receiving NAC were younger ($p = 0.051$), and more likely had downstaging to non-muscle invasive disease (10.7% versus 4.3%, $p = 0.042$). Median OS was 26.6 months. NAC patients had poorer OS compared with those who did receive NAC (Hazard ratio (HR) 1.6; $p = 0.019$). The persistence of muscle-invasive bladder in RC specimens was also significantly associated with OS (HR 2.40). In the NAC cohort, the two factors independently correlated with OS were the number of positive lymph nodes ($p = 0.013$) and adjuvant chemotherapy (AC) (HR 0.31; $p = 0.015$). Conclusions: Persistent nodal disease in RC specimens after NAC was associated with poor prognosis and lower OS rates compared with pN1-3 disease after upfront RC. In this sub-group of NAC patients, AC was independently associated with better OS.

Keywords: bladder cancer; nodal disease; pN1; radical cystectomy; neoadjuvant; adjuvant; chemotherapy

1. Introduction

Muscle-invasive bladder cancer is a highly aggressive disease with poor oncologic outcomes in case of lymph node involvement. Neoadjuvant chemotherapy (NAC) prior to radical cystectomy

(RC) has proven to improve survival outcomes in localized muscle-invasive bladder [1–3]. Level I evidence demonstrates a survival advantage of 5% as well as complete response on both primary and nodal tumor tissues [3]. The pN0 rate after NAC in cN+ patients has been evaluated as high as 48% in a retrospective series of 304 patients [4]. However, in spite of this proven overall survival (OS) advantage, a certain proportion of patients did not respond to NAC and exhibited aggressive patterns at the time of deferred RC, including pN1-3 disease. Despite NAC, up to one-fifth of the patients harbored nodal disease involvement at the time of RC [5]. However, the differential outcomes of pN1-3 patients stratified by the use or not of NAC is not well established. Moreover, there is little evidence and no firm recommendation on how to treat patients with positive lymph nodes after RC, especially after NAC administration [6]. In that setting, the use of adjuvant chemotherapy (AC) and of platinum-based regimens could be limited by potential tumor cells resistance and cumulative toxicity. Thus, whereas the impact of NAC on survival outcomes of cN1-3 patients prior to RC has been assessed in retrospective trials, to our knowledge, no series has compared OS between NAC and non-NAC patients harboring pN1-3 disease at the time of RC, and therefore the potential benefit of AC administration in that setting [4,7]. Studies comparing oncologic outcomes of pN1-3 disease according to the NAC status are biased by the selection, in the NAC group, of patients who did not respond to chemotherapy given persistent or progressing node disease after NAC. This selection bias based on resistance to neoadjuvant therapy has to be considered but helped to understand the need for aggressive post-RC treatment or monitoring in case of NAC failure.

2. Materials and Methods

2.1. Patients

We included 450 consecutive patients that underwent radical cystectomy (RC) for muscle-invasive urothelial bladder cancer with pathologically proven nodal disease from 2010 to 2019 at two institutions. After institutional review board approval (IRB number: 00006477 2017-016; review board: CEERB Paris Nord), all patients gave their written informed consent to participate in the prospective assessment of the outcomes (personal data collection and analysis). All RC were planned for cT2-4 cM0 disease, and we only included patients with pN1-3 disease. Clinical stage showed cT3 and cT4 disease in 31% and 20% of NAC patients, and 30% and 13.8% of non-NAC patients, respectively (48.2% of missing data for that variable). Patients with distant metastases (pM1a-b) on the pre-operative computerized tomography (CT) scan were excluded from analysis. The CT scan was systematically performed at the time of diagnosis. RC was performed less than 6 weeks after the diagnosis or less than 6 weeks after the last cycle of NAC. In case of NAC, another CT scan was performed before RC to confirm the absence of progression during NAC which would contra-indicate surgery. NAC and AC consisted of platinum-based chemotherapy. All patients treated by NAC received MVAC (methotrexate-vinblastine-doxorubicine-cisplatin) or GC (gemcitabline-cisplatin) regimen. AC was defined as a chemotherapy regimen given after RC before any sign of post-surgery progression, and platinum-based chemotherapy was the regimen of choice in the absence of contra-indication. Chemotherapy regimen and number of cycles were administered at clinician discretion in accordance with institutional standards and on individual decision-making. Patients treated with adjuvant radiotherapy or a combination of radiation and chemotherapy were excluded. All pathology data, including TNM stage, tumor grade, presence of positive soft tissue margin, total number of removed lymph nodes (LN), and number of LN+ were obtained from the pathological reports. Clinicopathological characteristics, surgical and adjuvant treatments, and follow-up data were collected in medical records. The chemotherapy status (NAC, AC) was recorded.

2.2. Primary and Secondary Endpoints and Statistics

The primary endpoint was the comparison between NAC and non-NAC in terms of death from any cause. Overall survival (OS) was assessed from the date of surgery until the date of death. OS was estimated using the Kaplan–Meier method and was compared using log-rank analysis OS rates were calculated with 95% confidence intervals. Multivariate Cox proportional hazards regression was used to estimate adjusted hazard ratios with 95% confidence interval. The limit of statistical significance was defined as $p < 0.05$. The SPSS 22.0 (IBM, Chicago, IL, USA) software was used for analysis.

3. Results

3.1. Clinical and Pathological Features of the Entire Cohort (n = 450)

Median age was 69 years with 73.1% male patients (Table 1). Downstaging to non-muscle invasive disease in RC specimens was 5.0%. Lymphovascular invasion and concomitant carcinoma in situ (CIS) were reported in 67.1% and 40.2% of cases, respectively. Soft tissue surgical margins were positive in 12.9% of the specimens. Median lymph node yield and positive lymph nodes were 16 and 2, respectively. Overall, 12.4% and 54.2% of patients received NAC +/− AC, and AC only, respectively. Among the overall cohort, 4.4% of patients received both chemo regimens. Approximately, half of patients died after a mean follow-up of 23 months. Distant systemic progression (bone and/or visceral metastases) was reported in 41.8% of patients.

Table 1. Overall cohort clinical and pathological characteristics ($n = 450$).

	N = 450
Gender (n, %):	
Male	329 (73.1)
Female	121 (26.9)
Age (years):	
Mean	67.5
Median (range) IQR	69.0 (25–93)
Pathological stage (n, %):	
pT0-pTis	12 (2.6)
pT1	11 (2.4)
pT2	78 (17.3)
pT3	247 (54.9)
pT4	102 (22.7)
Presence of lymphovascular invasion (n, %)	302 (67.1)
Presence of concomitant CIS (n, %)	181 (40.2)
Presence of soft tissue surgical margins (n, %)	58 (12.9)
Number of lymph nodes analyzed:	
Mean	17.5
Median (range) IQR	16.0 (1–70)
Number of positive lymph nodes:	
Mean	3.9
Median (range) IQR	2.0 (1–41)
Type of chemotherapy regimen (%):	
None	170 (37.8)
Neoadjuvant without adjuvant	36 (8.0)
Neoadjuvant + adjuvant	20 (4.4)
Adjuvant only	224 (54.2)
All-cause death (%)	220 (48.9)
Follow-up (months):	
Mean	23.0
Median (range) IQR	17.3 (3–130)

IQR = interquartile range, CIS = carcinoma in situ.

3.2. Comparisons of Clinical and Pathological Features Stratified by NAC Administration

Clinical and pathological features of both cohorts were compared (Table 2). Patients receiving NAC were younger (65 versus 68 years, $p = 0.051$), and more likely had downstaging to non-muscle invasive disease (10.7% versus 4.3%, $p = 0.042$). No significant difference was seen regarding CIS, lymphovascular invasion, positive lymph nodes, and soft tissue margin. Non-NAC patients were more frequently treated by AC (56.9% versus 35.7%, $p = 0.003$) and developed fewer systemic progression (39.1% versus 60.1%, $p = 0.002$).

Table 2. Comparisons between neoadjuvant chemotherapy (NAC) and non-NAC patients.

	NAC Cohort $N = 56$	Non-NAC Cohort $N = 394$	p-Value
Male (%) gender	46 (82.1)	283 (71.8)	0.103
Age (mean)	65.0	68.0	0.051
Pathological stage (%):			
pT0-pTis	3 (5.4)	9 (2.3)	
pT1	3 (5.4)	8 (2.0)	
pT2	6 (10.7)	72 (18.3)	0.097
pT3	29 (51.8)	218 (55.3)	
pT4	15 (26.8)	87 (22.1)	
Previous history of non-muscle-invasive bladder tumor before T2-4 diagnosis (%)	6 (10.7)	17 (4.3)	0.042
Presence of lymphovascular invasion (%)	42 (75.0)	260 (66.0)	0.179
Presence of concomitant CIS (%)	17 (30.4)	164 (41.6)	0.108
Soft tissue surgical margins (%)	7 (12.5)	51 (12.9)	0.926
Number of lymph nodes analyzed yield (mean)	17.6	17.1	0.777
Number of positive lymph nodes (mean)	3.8	4.8	0.197
Adjuvant chemotherapy administration (%)	20 (35.7)	224 (56.9)	0.003
Distant metastases (%)	34 (60.7)	154 (39.1)	0.002

NAC = neoadjuvant chemotherapy, CIS = carcinoma in situ.

3.3. Survival Analysis in the Overall Cohort

The OS curve of the overall cohort is shown in Figure 1A. Median OS was 26.6 months. The 1-, 2-, and 5-year OS rates were 75.9% (±2.1), 54.3% (±2.7), and 29.2% (±3.2) in the overall cohort.

NAC patients had poorer OS compared with those who did not receive NAC (log rank test: $p = 0.019$, Figure 1B). The 1-, 2-, and 5-year OS rates were 66.8% (±7.3), 34.6% (±8.3), and 16.3% (±7.7) in the NAC cohort, versus 76.9% (±2.2), 56.3% (±2.8), and 30.5% (±3.5) in the non-NAC cohort. Median OS in the NAC and non-NAC cohorts was 16.7 and 28.8 months, respectively.

The OS curves were then stratified according to the type of primary chemotherapy received (Figure 1C): no chemotherapy, NAC, or AC. Patients treated by AC had better OS outcomes compared with those receiving NAC or no chemotherapy (log rank test: $p < 0.001$). Median OS was 33.6 months, compared with 22.0 and 16.7 months in the no chemotherapy and NAC cohorts, respectively. Survival curves did not differ significantly between patients who did not receive any chemotherapy and NAC patients, in spite of a trend toward better outcomes during the first 18 months after RC ($p = 0.557$). Curves crossed at this time point with better long-term outcomes in patients without any neoadjuvant or adjuvant chemotherapy regimens.

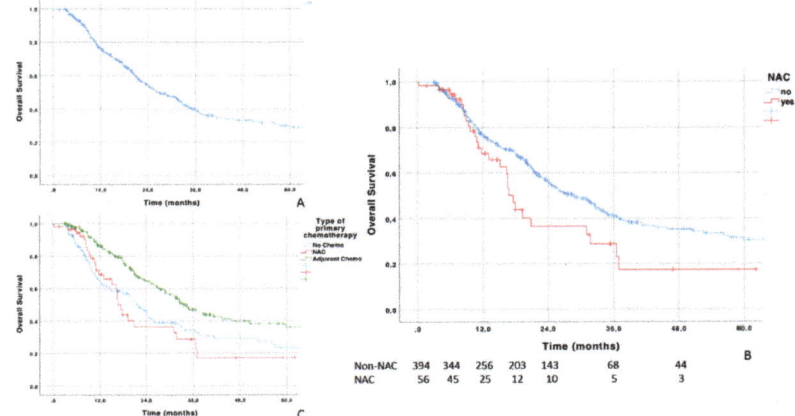

Figure 1. (**A**) Overall survival (OS) curve in the overall cohort; (**B**) OS stratified by the use of neoadjuvant chemotherapy (NAC); (**C**) OS stratified by the type of primary chemotherapy: neoadjuvant chemotherapy (NAC), adjuvant chemotherapy (AC), no chemotherapy.

3.4. Multivariable Analysis of Predictive Factors for OS in the Overall Cohort

Cox regression model confirmed that NAC was independently associated with overall mortality (Table 3). NAC patients had a 1.6-fold higher risk of death compared with non-NAC patients ($p = 0.018$; 95% confidence interval: 1.09–2.47). The persistence of muscle-invasive bladder in RC specimens was also significantly associated with OS (HR 2.40; 95% confidence interval: 1.06–5.44) This negative effect of NAC ($p = 0.072$) failed to reach significance when AC was taken into the multivariable model. AC was then positively and independently correlated with improved OS (HR 0.56; 95% confidence interval: 0.42–0.73; $p < 0.001$).

Table 3. Multivariable Cox regression analyses for predictors of overall survival (OS) in the overall cohort and in the neoadjuvant chemotherapy (NAC) cohort.

	HR	95% CI	*p*-Value
Overall cohort			
Model 1			
Gender	0.884	0.647–1.209	0.441
Age (continuous)	1.009	0.996–1.023	0.178
Muscle-invasive disease	2.404	1.062–5.442	0.035
Lymphovascular invasion	0.882	0.664–1.171	0.385
Concomitant CIS	1.088	0.830–1.427	0.540
Soft tissue surgical margin	1.338	0.910–1.965	0.138
Positive lymph nodes >3	1.283	0.959–1.717	0.093
NAC	1.638	1.089–2.465	0.018
Model 2			
NAC	1.445	0.968–2.159	0.072
Adjuvant Chemotherapy	0.557	0.426–0.728	<0.001
NAC cohort			
Muscle-invasive disease	0.296	0.060–1.470	0.137
Positive lymph nodes >3	3.281	1.287–8.365	0.013
Adjuvant chemotherapy	0.310	0.120–0.800	0.015

HR = hazard ratio; CI = confidence interval; CIS = carcinoma in situ.

3.5. Stratified Survival Analysis in NAC Cohort

Among NAC cohort, the administration of adjuvant chemotherapy was correlated with improved OS, without significant difference (Figure 2; $p = 0.099$). Median OS was 16.5 versus 31.7 months in patients receiving AC after NAC. The one-year OS rates were 61.9% (±9.7) versus 75.0% (±10.8) comparing patients who received AC and those who did not.

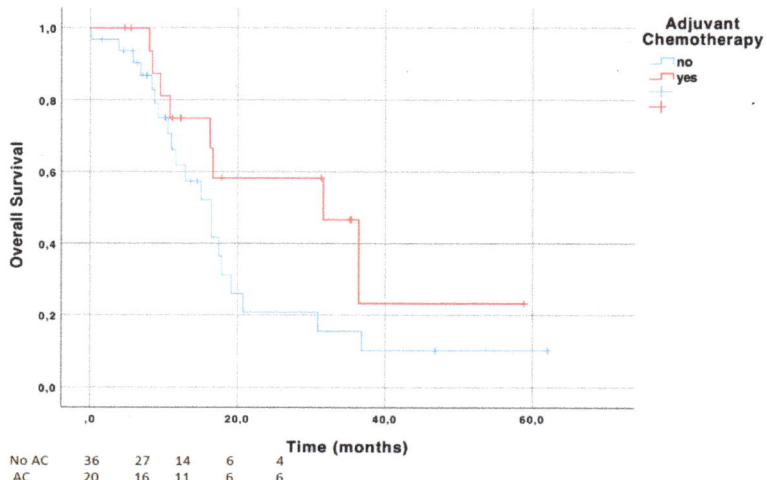

Figure 2. Survival curves for overall survival (OS) in the neoadjuvant chemotherapy (NAC) cohort stratified by the use of adjuvant chemotherapy (AC).

3.6. Multivariable Analysis of Factors Associated with Overall Mortality in the NAC Cohort

Cox regression analysis was performed in the subgroup of NAC patients (Table 3). Given the low number of patients ($n = 56$) and consequently the low number of events, we only included three factors which were the most correlated with overall mortality in univariable analyses. In the NAC cohort, the two factors independently correlated with overall mortality were the number of positive lymph nodes (>3 nodes; $p = 0.013$) and the administration of AC. AC was independently associated with a lower risk of overall mortality (HR 0.31; 95% confidence interval: 0.12–0.80; $p = 0.015$).

4. Discussion

NAC prior to RC has proven to improve survival outcomes in localized and locally advanced muscle-invasive bladder [1–3]. However, a non-negligible proportion of patients did not respond to NAC and exhibited aggressive patterns at the time of deferred RC including one-fifth of patients with nodal disease [5].

To date, there is little evidence on how to treat patients with positive lymph nodes after NAC and RC [6]. In a recent UK survey, 45% of oncologist responders would not give AC in patients with node disease after NAC and RC. Due to several factors, such as post-operative complications, impaired renal function, and poor performance status, the delivery of AC may be challenging even if an OS benefit is achieved [8]. Thus, the feasibility of re-challenging this group of NAC patients with AC is currently not well established, and patients are often offered salvage chemotherapy only at time of disease progression for palliation. A previous study of 37 patients with node positive disease after NAC previously suggested that patients who have persistent nodal disease have a very poor prognosis [9]. The two-year OS survival rate was 20%. The findings of this single-arm retrospective study highlighted a potential benefit from adjuvant chemotherapy. As reported in our series, there was a trend toward improved OS when AC was used.

While the rate of pT0 disease after NAC has been well assessed in the literature (approximately 30%), the complete response rate in node cannot be accurately evaluated due to the inaccuracy of preoperative evaluation. Indeed, node staging is currently performed by CT scan or pelvic magnetic resonance imaging (MRI). Both procedures are limited by poor sensitivity and specificity. In a series of clinical node-positive patients prior to NAC, Hermans et al. suggested that the rate of complete post-NAC response in pelvic lymph nodes (pN0) was 31% and 19% in cN1 and cN2-3 patients, respectively [7]. A complete response in lymph nodes has been evaluated at 48% in another retrospective study [4]. We were unable to assess this node downstaging rate given that we only included pN1-3 patients. However, even in patients having an aggressive disease with positive nodes at RC, our study suggests a positive impact of NAC on tumor tissue given that the pT0-1 rate was 10.8% in the NAC cohort, versus 4.3% only in non-NAC patients ($p = 0.042$). Unfortunately, given the limitations already evoked, the potential difference of response between primary cancer and metastatic nodal tissue cannot be relevantly evaluated.

The poorer OS achieved by NAC versus non-NAC patients with pN1-3 disease confirmed the need for adapting post-RC treatment in this high-risk sub-population. These patients will more frequently develop post-RC systemic progression (60.7% versus 39.1%) and die prematurely. Our findings suggest that the use of AC could be beneficial even after NAC. Indeed, OS was improved when AC was given, and AC was an independent protective factor in multivariable analysis, after taking into account positive lymph node burden and pT stage.

Consistently with French habits, MVAC was regarded in our experience as the first-line treatment of choice [10]. The pathological complete response rate achieved by dose dense MVAC appeared better than GC in retrospective studies [11]. Few patients received GC which could be preferred in other centers and/or countries due to a better toxicity profile. Comparable efficacy of GC has been emphasized, but in the metastatic setting [12]. Preliminary data from the VESPER trial (NCT01812369), comparing GC and MVAC as NAC, were presented recently, and the mature publication is awaited.

The role of AC after RC remains controversial. The main data come from underpowered trials due to poor recruitment, or from studies suffering from methodological issues. The advent of NAC before RC has also had a negative impact on enrollment in such trials [13]. The European Organisation for Research and Treatment of Cancer (NCT 30994) evaluated four cycles of immediate adjuvant chemotherapy versus six cycles of deferred chemotherapy at the time of relapse [14]. The benefit in OS was only seen in a small sub-group of pN0 patients ($n = 86$). Meta-analyses tend to confirm the reduction in the risk of death with AC (approximately 23%) [15,16]. Thus, although AC is no longer recommended, evidence suggests that it could be efficient, but mainly in chemotherapy-naive patients with locally advanced bladder cancer (pT3-4, pN0/pN +, pM0). Until now, no prospective trial has compared the sequence NAC versus NAC plus AC in patients with persistent locally advanced bladder cancer or lymph node involvement at the time of RC.

We did not report the detailed chemotherapy regimens in terms of number of cycles, toxicity data, palliative chemotherapy, and number of subsequent lines. The OS we showed could be impacted by all these parameters. Subsequent therapies for metastatic disease, that may have affected OS rates, were not available for all patients. Until recently, the only licensed second-line chemotherapy was vinflunine, which has demonstrated a three-month survival benefit with toxicity. However, the therapy landscape of advanced bladder cancer rapidly evolves. It is also worthy to note that this cohort was followed before the approval of immunotherapy regimens in advanced bladder cancer. The implementation of immunotherapy in the metastatic as well as in the neoadjuvant setting may modify the response to neoadjuvant treatment, as well as progression-free and overall survival [17]. In this study, we found that NAC patients treated by AC after RC achieved better OS outcomes compared with patients receiving only palliative chemotherapy. However, only one-third of NAC patients received AC due to poor performance status, post-operative complications, cumulative toxicity or various reasons.

The possibility to change AC for adjuvant immunotherapy could increase the number of NAC patients eligible for adjuvant therapy and offer life-prolonging drug options in that particular setting of pN1-3 NAC patients.

The combination of therapy could also be an interesting option in pN1-3 disease. Zaghloul et al. recently demonstrated in a phase II study that the addition of radiotherapy to AC could improve the locoregional recurrence-free survival [18]. The trend reported in terms of OS has to be confirmed in larger phase III trials. The GETUG-AFU 30 trial (NCT03333356) is ongoing to evaluate the benefit of adjuvant radiotherapy in high-risk cancers in terms of pelvic recurrence-free survival as primary endpoint, and OS as secondary endpoint.

It seemed worthy to note that we only included in this study NAC patients who did not respond to chemotherapy given persistent or progressing node disease after NAC. This sub-group selection based on first therapy resistance explained the worse prognosis of NAC patients compared with non-NAC patients who were not selected by any type of treatment resistance. This selection bias has to be considered and helps to understand the need for aggressive post-RC treatment or monitoring in case of NAC failure.

Finally, the main limitation was the difficulty to draw any firm conclusion based on a retrospective study. In addition to potential selection biases in the selection of patients for NAC, for surgery and for AC, our results could have also been limited by the relatively small sample size. Currently, it is not possible to establish with absolute certainty what is the best sequence of perioperative treatments. However, to our knowledge, this study was the first to directly compare contemporary outcomes after RC in pN1-3 patients treated or not with NAC, and it confirmed the potential of AC even in patients already treated by NAC.

5. Conclusions

Persistent nodal disease in RC specimens after NAC is associated with poor prognosis and lower OS rates compared with pN1-3 disease after upfront RC. In this sub-group of NAC patients, AC was given to one-third of NAC patients and was an independent predictive factor for better OS outcomes. Larger prospective data as well as studies assessing the impact of other adjuvant therapies such as immunotherapy or radiotherapy are awaited.

Author Contributions: Conceptualization, G.P. and M.R.; data curation, G.P., B.P., J.-B.B., A.-P.L., A.S., E.X., and D.P.; formal analysis, G.P., B.P., J.-B.B., C.C., C.A., E.S., J.-R.G., M.R., C.T., L.M., A.S., E.X., and D.P.; investigation, J.-B.B., E.S., and G.L.; methodology, B.P., J.-B.B., J.-R.G., and G.L.; supervision, C.C., A.-P.L., G.L., C.T., and L.M.; validation, C.C., C.A., E.S., J.-R.G., A.-P.L., M.R., G.L., C.T., L.M., A.S., E.X., and D.P.; visualization, C.A.; writing—original draft, G.P., B.P., E.X., and D.P.; writing—review and editing, C.C., C.A., E.S., J.-R.G., A.-P.L., M.R., C.T., L.M., and A.S. All authors have read and agreed to the published version of the manuscript.

Funding: This research received no external funding.

Conflicts of Interest: The authors declare no conflict of interest.

References

1. Griffiths, G.; Hall, R.; Sylvester, R.; Raghavan, D.; Parmar, M.K.; Club Urologico Espanol de Tratamiento Oncologico Group. International phase III trial assessing neoadjuvant cisplatin, methotrexate, and vinblastine chemotherapy for muscle-invasive bladder cancer: Longterm results of the BA06 30894 trial. *J. Clin. Oncol.* **2011**, *29*, 2171. [PubMed]
2. Grossman, H.B.; Natale, R.B.; Tangen, C.M.; Speights, V.O.; Vogelzang, N.J.; Trump, D.L.; White, R.W.D.; Sarosdy, M.F.; Wood, D.P., Jr.; Raghavan, D.; et al. Neoadjuvant chemotherapy plus cystectomy compared with cystectomy alone for locally advanced bladder cancer. *N. Engl. J. Med.* **2003**, *349*, 859–866. [CrossRef] [PubMed]

3. Vale, C.L.; Advanced Bladder Cancer (ABC) Meta-analysis Collaboration. Neoadjuvant chemotherapy in invasive bladder cancer: Update of a systematic review and meta-analysis of individual patient data advanced bladder cancer (ABC) meta analysis collaboration. *Eur. Urol.* **2005**, *48*, 202–206. [CrossRef] [PubMed]
4. Zargar-Shoshtari, K.; Zargar, H.; Lotan, Y.; Shah, J.B.; van Rhijn, B.W.; Daneshmand, S.; Spiess, P.E.; Black, P.C.; Fairey, L.S.M.C.A.S.; Fairey, A.S.; et al. A Multi-Institutional Analysis of Outcomes of Patients with Clinically Node Positive Urothelial Bladder Cancer Treated with Induction Chemotherapy and Radical Cystectomy. *J. Urol.* **2016**, *195*, 53–59. [CrossRef]
5. Mertens, L.S.; Meijer, R.P.; Meinhardt, W.; Van Der Poel, H.G.; Bex, A.; Kerst, J.M.; Van Der Heijden, M.S.; Bergman, A.M.; Horenblas, S.; Van Rhijn, B.W.G. Occult lymph node metastases in patients with carcinoma invading bladder muscle: Incidence after neoadjuvant chemotherapy and cystectomy vs. after cystectomy alone. *BJU Int.* **2014**, *114*, 67–74. [CrossRef] [PubMed]
6. Tan, W.S.; Lamb, B.W.; Payne, H.; Hughes, S.; Green, J.S.; Lane, T.; Adshead, J.; Boustead, G.; Vasdev, N. Management of Node-Positive Bladder Cancer after Neoadjuvant Chemotherapy and Radical Cystectomy: A Survey of Current UK Practice. *Clin. Genitourin. Cancer* **2015**, *13*, e153–e158. [CrossRef] [PubMed]
7. Hermans, T.J.; van de Putte, E.E.F.; Horenblas, S.; Meijer, R.P.; Boormans, J.L.; Aben, K.K.H.; Van Der Heijden, M.S.; De Wit, R.; Beerepoot, L.V.; Verhoeven, R.; et al. Pathological downstaging and survival after induction chemotherapy and radical cystectomy for clinically node-positive bladder cancer-Results of a nationwide population-based study. *Eur. J. Cancer* **2016**, *69*, 1–8. [CrossRef] [PubMed]
8. Herr, H.W.; Dotan, Z.; Donat, S.M.; Bajorin, D.F. Defining optimal therapy for muscle invasive bladder cancer. *J. Urol.* **2007**, *177*, 437–443. [CrossRef] [PubMed]
9. Kassouf, W.; Agarwal, P.K.; Grossman, H.B.; Leibovici, D.; Munsell, M.F.; Siefker-Radtke, A.; Pisters, L.L.; Swanson, D.A.; Dinney, C.P.N.; Kamatbe, A.M. Outcome of patients with bladder cancer with pN♭ disease after preoperative chemotherapy and radical cystectomy. *Urology* **2009**, *73*, 147–152. [CrossRef] [PubMed]
10. Zargar, H.; Shah, J.B.; van Rhijn, B.W.; Daneshmand, S.; Bivalacqua, T.J.; Spiess, P.E.; Black, P.C.; Kassouf, W.; Van De Putte, E.E.F.; Horenblas, S.; et al. Neoadjuvant Dose Dense MVAC versus Gemcitabine and Cisplatin in Patients with cT3-4aN0M0 Bladder Cancer Treated with Radical Cystectomy. *J. Urol.* **2018**, *199*, 1452–1458. [CrossRef] [PubMed]
11. Loehrer, P.J.; Einhorn, L.H.; Elson, P.J.; Crawford, E.D.; Kuebler, P.; Tannock, I.; Raghavan, D. Stuart-Harris, R.; Sarosdy, M.F.; Lowe, B.A. A randomized comparison of cisplatin alone or in combination with methotrexate, vinblastine, and doxorubicin in patients with metastatic urothelial carcinoma: A cooperative group study. *J. Clin. Oncol.* **1992**, *10*, 1066–1073. [CrossRef] [PubMed]
12. von der Maase, H.; Hansen, S.W.; Roberts, J.T.; Dogliotti, L.; Oliver, T.; Moore, M.; Bodrogi, I.; Albers, P.; Knuth, A.; Lippert, C.; et al. Gemcitabine and cisplatin versus methotrexate, vinblastine, doxorubicin, and cisplatin in advanced or metastatic bladder cancer: Results of a large, randomized, multinational, multicenter, phase III study. *J. Clin. Oncol.* **2000**, *18*, 3068–3077. [CrossRef] [PubMed]
13. Paz-Ares, L.; Solsona, E.; Esteban, E.; Saez, A.; Gonzalez-Larriba, J.; Anton, A.; de la Rosa, F.; Guillem, V.; Bellmunt, J. On behalf of the SOGUG and GUO-AEU groups Randomized phase III trial comparing adjuvant paclitaxel/gemcitabine/cisplatin (PGC to observation in patients with resected invasive bladder cancer: Results of the SOGUG (Spanish Oncology Genito-Urinary Group) 99/01 study. *J. Clin. Oncol.* **2010**, *4518*. [CrossRef]
14. Sternberg, C.N.; Skoneczna, I.; Kerst, J.M.; Albers, P.; Fossa, S.D.; Agerbaek, M.; Dumez, H.; de Santis, M.; Théodore, C.; Leahy, M.G.; et al. Immediate versus deferred chemotherapy after radical cystectomy in patients with pT3-pT4 or N1M0 urothelial carcinoma of the bladder (EORTC 30994): An intergroup, open-label, randomised phase 3 trial. *Lancet Oncol.* **2015**, *16*, 76–86. [CrossRef]
15. Leow, J.J.; Martin-Doyle, W.; Rajagopal, P.S.; Patel, C.G.; Anderson, E.M.; Rothman, A.T.; Cote, R.J.; Urun, Y.; Chang, S.L.; Choueiri, T.K.; et al. Adjuvant chemotherapy for invasive bladder cancer: A 2013 updated systematic review and meta-analysis of randomized trials. *Eur. Urol.* **2014**, *66*, 42–54. [CrossRef] [PubMed]
16. Wosnitzer, M.S.; Hruby, G.W.; Murphy, A.M.; Barlow, L.J.; Cordon-Cardo, C.; Mansukhani, M.; Petrylak, D.P.; Benson, M.C.; McKiernan, J.M.; Cordon-Cardo, C. A comparison of the outcomes of neoadjuvant and adjuvant chemotherapy for clinical T2-T4aN0-N2M0 bladder cancer. *Cancer* **2012**, *118*, 353–364. [CrossRef] [PubMed]

17. Necchi, A.; Anichini, A.; Raggi, D.; Briganti, A.; Massa, S.; Lucianò, R.; Colecchia, M.; Giannatempo, P.; Mortarini, R.; Bianchi, M.; et al. Pembrolizumab as Neoadjuvant Therapy Before Radical Cystectomy in Patients With Muscle-Invasive Urothelial Bladder Carcinoma (PURE-01): An Open-Label, Single-Arm, Phase II Study. *J. Clin. Oncol.* **2018**, *20*, 3353–3360. [CrossRef] [PubMed]
18. Zaghloul, M.S.; Christodouleas, J.P.; Smith, A.; Abdallah, A.; William, H.; Khaled, H.M.; Hwang, W.-T.; Baumann, B.C. Adjuvant sandwich chemotherapy plus radiotherapy vs. adjuvant chemotherapy alone for locally advanced bladder cancer after radical cystectomy. A randomized phase 2 trial. *JAMA Surg.* **2018**, *153*, e174591. [CrossRef] [PubMed]

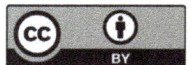

© 2020 by the authors. Licensee MDPI, Basel, Switzerland. This article is an open access article distributed under the terms and conditions of the Creative Commons Attribution (CC BY) license (http://creativecommons.org/licenses/by/4.0/).

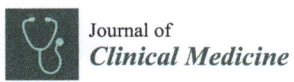

Article

Differential Expression and Clinicopathological Significance of HER2, Indoleamine 2,3-Dioxygenase and PD-L1 in Urothelial Carcinoma of the Bladder

Donghyun Kim [1,2], Jin Man Kim [1,2], Jun-Sang Kim [3,4], Sup Kim [4,*] and Kyung-Hee Kim [1,2,5,*]

1. Department of Pathology, Chungnam National University School of Medicine, 266 Munhwa Street, Daejeon 35015, Korea; duras3516@cnuh.co.kr (D.K.); jinmank@cnu.ac.kr (J.M.K.)
2. Department of Pathology, Chungnam National University Hospital, 282 Munwha-ro, Daejeon 35015, Korea
3. Department of Radiation Oncology, Chungnam National University School of Medicine, 288 Munhwa Street, Daejeon 35015, Korea; k423j@cnu.ac.kr
4. Department of Radiation Oncology, Chungnam National University Hospital, 282 Munwha-ro, Daejeon 35015, Korea
5. Department of Pathology, Chungnam National University Sejong Hospital, 20 Bodeum 7-ro, Sejong-si 30099, Korea
* Correspondence: supkim@cnuh.co.kr (S.K.); phone330@cnu.ac.kr (K.-H.K.); Tel.: +82-42-280-7860 (S.K.); +82-42-580-8238 (K.-H.K.); Fax: +82-42-280-7899 (S.K.); +82-42-280-7189 (K.-H.K.)

Received: 6 March 2020; Accepted: 24 April 2020; Published: 27 April 2020

Abstract: Purpose: Evasion of the immune system by cancer cells allows for the progression of tumors. Antitumor immunotherapy has shown remarkable effects in a diverse range of cancers. The aim of this study was to determine the clinicopathological significance of human epidermal growth factor receptor 2 (HER2), indoleamine 2,3-dioxygenase (IDO), and programmed death ligand-1 (PD-L1) expression in urothelial carcinoma of the bladder (UCB). Materials and Methods: We retrospectively studied 97 patients with UCB. We performed an immunohistochemical study to measure the expression levels of HER2, IDO, and PD-L1 in UCB tissue from these 97 patients. Results: In all 97 cases, the PD-L1 expression of tumor-infiltrating immune cells (ICs) was significantly correlated with higher pathologic tumor stage (pT). In pT2–pT4 cases ($n = 69$), higher levels of HER2 and IDO expression in invasive tumor cells (TCs) were associated with shorter periods of disease-free survival (DFS). Conclusion: These results imply that the expression of PD-L1 in ICs of the UCB microenvironment is associated with cancer invasion and the expression of HER2 or IDO in the invasive cancer cell and suggestive of the potential for cancer recurrence. We suggest that the expression levels of IDO, HER2, and PD-L1 could be useful as targets in the development of combined cancer immunotherapeutic strategies.

Keywords: human epidermal growth factor receptor 2; indoleamine 2,3-dioxygenase; programmed death ligand-1; urothelial carcinoma; urinary bladder; immunotherapy

1. Introduction

Urothelial carcinoma of the bladder (UCB) remains one of the most common malignant cancers of the genitourinary tract [1]. Among UCB patients, approximately 30% will have muscle invasion at diagnosis, show rapid progression to metastatic disease, and succumb to their disease [2]. Although there are several different treatment regimens, very poor treatment outcomes have been reported in locally advanced and metastatic UCB patients, and this trend has remained unchanged in the last few decades [3,4]. Therefore, further studies are required to better understand the molecular mechanisms of tumor aggressiveness in UCB.

One barrier limiting the efficacy of classic cancer therapies is the interactions of cancer cells with their microenvironment, which ultimately determine whether the primary tumor is eradicated, metastasizes, or establishes dormant micrometastases [5]. Furthermore, the tumor microenvironment can also determine treatment outcome and resistance [6]. Thus, future anticancer treatment strategies should not only act directly on the proliferative processes of transformed cells but also interrupt the crosstalk circuits established by tumor cells with the host microenvironment [7].

Tumor immunogenicity is simply defined as the ability to induce adaptive immune responses [6]. Although most tumors carry particular substances which can induce an immune response, such as antigens or epitopes, the immunogenicity of cancer varies greatly between cancer types. It has been reported that tumor immunogenicity relies on its own antigenicity and several immunomodulatory mechanisms that render tumor cells less sensitive to immune system attack, or create a highly immunosuppressive tumor microenvironment [8]. Classic cancer therapies, such as chemotherapy and radiotherapy, reduce the tumor burden by killing cancer cells. Furthermore, during apoptosis and necrosis, antigens and damage-associated molecular patterns (DAMPs) stimulate an antitumor immune response which induces immunogenic cell death [9,10]. However, cancer cells can escape immune surveillance and progress through modulating immune checkpoint molecules that suppress antitumor immune responses [8].

Considering their high immunogenicity, the expression levels of immune checkpoint-related proteins have been measured and linked to the clinicopathological features and treatment outcomes in UCB. Many studies have reported that expression of immune checkpoint-related proteins, such as programmed cell death 1 (PD-1)/programmed death ligand-1 (PD-L1) and indoleamine 2,3-dioxygenase (IDO) show prognostic significance in UCB [11–13]. Additionally, various cancers have responded to treatment with immune checkpoint inhibitors, including UCB [14].

In breast cancer, Filippo et al. highlighted the role of innate and adaptive immune responses in HER2-targeted drugs [15]. This article has prompted investigations into the interaction of immune checkpoint proteins with HER2 targeted therapies. Recently, human epidermal growth factor receptor 2 (HER2) signals have been found to potentially regulate the infiltration of tumor microenvironment immune cells, and to have a role in the expression of PD-L1 in breast and gastric cancers [16,17]. Similarly, increased IDO expression was observed in a subset of HER2+ breast tumors (43.1%), which could be used to develop a combination treatment regimen [18]. These results suggest that immune-escape genes could be used to develop a combination treatment regimen in HER2 overexpression UCB patients. However, the clinical significance of immune checkpoint-related molecules in the context of HER2-positive and -negative UCB have not yet been fully evaluated.

We hypothesized that information on the expression of HER2 and immune-escape genes could be useful in the development of therapeutic strategies. This study aimed to evaluate the expression levels of HER2 and immune-escape genes by immunohistochemistry (IHC) in 97 cases of UCB. Therefore, we first evaluated the influence of immune cell infiltration on UCB survival using the Tumor IMmune Estimation Resource (TIMER) database. Then, to identify immunomodulatory genes, correlations between CD8+ T cell infiltration and candidate genes were analyzed by TIMER. Finally, we evaluated expression levels of HER2, IDO, and PD-L1 by immunohistochemistry (IHC) in 97 cases of UCB. The levels of these three protein expressions were correlated with various clinicopathological characteristics, including patient survival.

2. Patients and Methods

2.1. Patients and Tissue Samples

This study was approved by the Institutional Review Board of Chungnam National University Hospital (CNUH 2019-10-041). All formalin-fixed paraffin-embedded (FFPE) tissue samples for IHC and clinical data were obtained from the National Biobank of Korea at Chungnam National University Hospital. The requirement for informed consent for the retrospective comparison study was waived because the study was based on immunohistochemical analysis using FFPE tissue.

We conducted a review of the records of 97 patients with UCB between 1999 and 2014 at Chungnam National University Hospital in Daejeon, South Korea. The inclusion criteria were that the FFPE UCB tissues were available, and that the follow-up clinical data were sufficiently detailed. The exclusion criteria were as follows: (1) patients had a previous history of other cancers; (2) patients had received previous curative resection for any urinary tract tumor lesion; (3) patients had received preoperative chemotherapy or radiation therapy; or (4) patients had received any molecular targeted therapy. The tumor, node, and metastasis (TNM) staging and histologic grading for UCB were determined at the time of tumor resection, and were based on the 8th edition of the American Joint Committee on Cancer (AJCC) staging system [19].

The 97 UCB cases included 4 cases of noninvasive papillary urothelial carcinoma, 24 cases of pT1, 40 cases of pT2, 26 cases of pT3, and 3 cases of pT4. The 28 patients who underwent transurethral resection of the bladder (TUR-B) were in the pathologic tumor stage (pT) pTa–pT1; the 69 patients who underwent total or partial cystectomy were pT2–pT4. The histologic type of all 97 cases was conventional urothelial carcinoma. For the 69 cases of pT2–pT4, data were collected regarding their disease-free survival (DFS) and overall survival (OS) periods. Among the 69 cases, 29 patients underwent post-operative radiotherapy (PORT). DFS was determined as the time interval between the date of initial surgical resection and the date of UCB recurrence or metastasis. UCB recurrence or metastasis was determined via imaging and/or histological analysis. OS was defined as from the time of initial surgical resection to the date of death due to any cause. Without confirmation of death, recurrence, or metastasis, OS or DFS time was recorded based on the last known date that the patient was alive. We used representative FFPE whole-tissue samples of 97 UCB cases for immunohistochemistry (IHC).

2.2. Immunohistochemical Staining Analysis

Immunohistochemical staining of the FFPE tissue sample of UCB was conducted as previously described [20]. Target Retrieval Solution, pH 9 (catalog #S2368, Dako, Glostrup, Denmark), was used for antigen revitalization. The tissue sections were incubated for 30 min at room temperature with the following primary antibodies: rabbit polyclonal anti-human c-erbB-2 oncoprotein (1:200, catalog #A0485, Dako, Glostrup, Denmark), rabbit polyclonal anti-PD-L1 antibody (1:200, catalog #GTX104763, CD274 molecule, GeneTex, Irvine, CA, USA), mouse monoclonal anti-indoleamine 2,3-dioxygenase antibody, clone 10.1 (1:100, catalog #MAB5412, MERCK, Bellanca, MA, USA), CD8 (Ready-to-Use, catalog #IR623, Dako, Glostrup, Denmark), and CD43 (Ready-to-Use, catalog #IR636, Dako, Glostrup, Denmark).

We only scored HER2, IDO, and PD-L1 IHC stains for invasive urothelial carcinoma cells of 93 invasive UCB cases, while four cases of noninvasive papillary urothelial carcinoma were evaluated for intraepithelial dysplastic urothelial cells. We analyzed the cytoplasmic or cytoplasmic membrane expression of HER2 using the modified DAKO HercepTest ^{TM} Interpretation Manual—Breast Cancer Row version [21] (Staining scored 0, 1+, 2+ and 3+). Staining of 2+ or 3+ was regarded as high expression of HER2. The PD-L1 IHC staining was interpreted using the PD-L1 IHC 22C3 pharmDx Interpretation Manual—Urothelial Carcinoma [22] and VENTANA PD-L1 (SP142) Assay Interpretation Guide for Urothelial Carcinoma [23]. Any convincing partial or complete linear cytoplasmic membrane staining of viable tumor cells (TCs) exceeding 1% of the tumor cell proportion was defined as high expression of TC. Presence of discernible PD-L1, CD43, and CD8 staining of any intensity in the tumor-infiltrating immune cells (ICs) covering ≥1% of the tumor area was regarded as high expression of ICs. For CD43 and CD8, we only scored IHC staining of tumor microenvironment ICs in the muscularis propria of 61 cystectomized UCB cases among 67 cases of pT2–pT4. IDO cytoplasmic expression in TCs was scored using the method described by Allred et al. (score 0–8) [24]. A high expression of IDO was regarded as a median score or above (score ≥5). The results were examined separately and scored by Kim, K-H, and Kim, J-M, who were blinded to the patients' clinicopathological details. Any discrepancies in the scores were discussed to obtain a consensus.

2.3. TIMER Database Analysis

TIMER is a comprehensive resource for systematic analysis of immune infiltrates across diverse cancer types (https://cistrome.shinyapps.io/timer/) [25]. TIMER applies a deconvolution previously published statistical method to infer the abundance of tumor-infiltrating immune cells (TIICs) from gene expression profiles [26]. We investigated the relationship between tumor-infiltrating immune cells and UCB survival outcomes. Additionally, we analyzed the correlation of PDL1, IDO, CTLA4, CCL1, CCL2, and CCR2 expression with the abundance of CD8+ T cells.

2.4. Statistical Analyses

The correlations of the clinicopathological parameters with expressions of HER2, IDO, and PD-L1 were evaluated using Pearson's chi-square test and Fisher's exact test. The associations between HER2, IDO, PD-L1, CD43 and CD8 proteins were examined by Spearman rank correlation coefficients. Postoperative OS and DFS were determined using Kaplan–Meier survival curves and a log-rank test. The Cox proportional hazards model was applied for univariate and multivariate survival analyses. The mean values of absolute lymphocyte count (ALC), absolute neutrophil count (ANC), and neutrophil to lymphocyte ratio (NLR) were compared for the subgroups with HER2, IDO, PD-L1 (TCs), and PD-L1 (ICs) expression using an unpaired Student's t-test. Statistical significance was set at $p < 0.05$ (SPSS v.24; SPSS Inc., Chicago, IL, USA).

3. Results

3.1. Association of Immune Cell Infiltration with Survival and Expression of Immune Escape Genes

Even if there is evidence for the action of various immune cell populations in bladder cancer, a comprehensive landscape of the immune response to UCB and its driving forces is still lacking. Therefore, we tried to identify the correlation between immune cell infiltration of this cancer and survival by using the TIMER (Tumor IMmune Estimation Resource) database. In UCB, only the immune infiltrating level of CD8+ T cells was negatively correlated with survival (Figure S1). These results are in line with the tumorcidial function of CD8+ T in immune cells, which can be mitigated by the immune escape mechanism [27].

It was reported that various molecules may be involved in tumor-induced immune tolerance in UCB [28,29]. Therefore, we evaluated the correlation between CD8+ T cell infiltration of UCB and these molecules by using TIMER. Among various molecules, PD-L1 and IDO1 expression are most highly correlated with CD8+ T cell infiltration in UCB (Table S1).

3.2. Association of Clinicopathological Characteristics with Expression of HER2, IDO and PD-L1

The 97 UCB cases were evaluated using IHC to determine HER2, IDO, and PD-L1 levels. The clinicopathological characteristics of the 97 UCB patients associated with expressions of HER2, IDO, and PD-L1 are presented in Table 1. Most non-neoplastic urothelial epithelial cells or noninvasive urothelial carcinoma cells showed no expression of PD-L1, while HER2 and IDO were generally expressed with mild to moderate intensity in a large majority of reactive urothelial cells or noninvasive intraepithelial urothelial carcinoma cells, while there was no expression of IDO in normal urothelial epithelia. Invasive UCB cancer cells in lamina propria showed a relatively decreased expression of HER2 or IDO in comparison to the expression of reactive or dysplastic intraepithelial urothelial cells (Figure 1). Invasive UCB was scored using IHC stains of deeper invasive cancer lesions, except for intraepithelial lesion. However, the noninvasive papillary urothelial carcinomas were evaluated for intraepithelial dysplastic urothelial cells. Expression of HER2 or IDO in the 97 cases of UCB showed trends of decreased expression in pT2–pT4 compared to pTa–pT1 ($p = 0.055$ and $p = 0.0007$). However, PD-L1 expression of ICs was higher in pT2–pT4 than in pTa–pT1 ($p = 0.001$). HER2 expression in TCs was marginally associated with ALC /µL ($p = 0.069$). IDO expression in TCs was positively correlated with ALC /µL ($p = 0.030$) and was negatively correlated with ANC /µL ($p = 0.007$) and NLR ($p = 0.050$).

PD-L1 expression in ICs was positively correlated with ANC /µL ($p = 0.041$) and NLR ($p = 0.063$) (Table S2).

Table 1. Correlations of HER2, IDO, and PD-L1 expressions with clinicopathological factors in 97 patients with urothelial carcinoma of the bladder.

Variable	No.	HER2			IDO			PD-L1 (TCs)			PD-L1 (ICs)		
		Low	High	p *	Low	High	p *	Low	High	p *	Low	High	p *
Gender		$N=46$	$N=51$	0.605	$N=45$	$N=52$	0.676	$N=52$	$N=45$	0.102	$N=48$	$N=49$	0.760
Male	78	38	40		37	41		45	33		38	40	
Female	19	8	11		8	11		7	12		10	9	
Age (years)				0.087			0.164			0.900			0.732
≤65	36	13	23		20	16		19	17		17	19	
>65	61	33	28		25	36		33	28		31	30	
Grade				1.000			0.029			1.000			0.436
low	6	3	3		0	6		3	3		4	2	
high	91	43	48		45	46		49	42		44	47	
Tumor stage				0.055			0.007			0.179			0.001
pTa–pT1	28	9	19		7	21		18	10		21	7	
pT2–pT4	69	37	32		38	31		34	35		27	42	

* Pearson's chi-square test or Fisher's exact test.

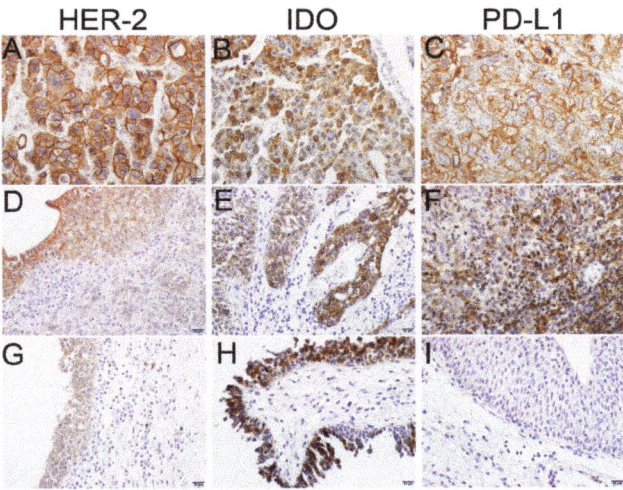

Figure 1. Representative images of HER2, IDO, and PD-L1 immunohistochemical staining in urothelial carcinoma of the bladder (UCB). (**A–C**) Invasive cancer cells with strongly positive expressions of HER2, IDO, and PD-L1. (**D**) Intermediate positive expression of HER2 in low-grade noninvasive urothelial tumor (left upper) and very weakly positive expression of HER2 in invasive cancer cells (right lower). (**E**) Intermediate positive expression of IDO in a low-grade noninvasive urothelial tumor (left) and strongly positive expression of IDO in a high-grade urothelial tumor (right). (**F**) Strongly positive expression of PD-L1 in intra-tumoral immune cells. (**G**) Weakly positive expression of HER2 in reactive urothelial epithelium. (**H**) Strongly positive in situ expression of IDO in urothelial carcinoma. (**I**) Negative expression of PD-L1 in reactive urothelium (scale bar = 20 µm).

3.3. Correlation Between Expression of HER2, IDO, PD-L1, CD43 and CD8 Measured in Tumor Cells or Immune Cells

The correlation between expression of the five proteins is presented in Table 2. CD43 is one of the major glycoproteins of thymocytes and T lymphocytes, suggesting a negative regulatory role in adaptive immune reactions as one of the positive markers of myeloid-derived suppressor cell phenotyping. The inverse correlation between PD-L1 expression in ICs and IDO expression in TCs was observed ($p = 0.010$). HER2 expression in TC was marginally associated with IDO expression in TCs ($p = 0.058$). There was significant positive correlation between the expression of PD-L1, CD43 and CD8 in ICs. There was a tendency to have a negative feedback phenomenon between the expression of IDO and HER2 in TC and the expression of PD-L1, CD43, and CD8 in ICs.

Table 2. Correlations between HER2, IDO, PD-L1, CD43, and CD8 expression according to immunohistochemical staining of urothelial carcinoma of the bladder.

Spearman's rho		HER2 (TCs)	IDO (TCs)	PD-L1 (TCs)	PD-L1 (ICs)	CD43 (ICs)	CD8 (ICs)
HER2 (TCs)	Correlation coefficient	1.000	0.193	−0.110	−0.155	−0.091	−0.021
	Sig. (2-tailed) *	-	0.058	0.283	0.129	0.485	0.875
	No.	97	97	97	97	61	61
IDO (TCs)	Correlation coefficient	0.193	1.000	−0.171	−0.259 *	−0.247	−0.126
	Sig. (2-tailed) *	0.058	-	0.094	0.010	0.055	0.334
	No.	97	97	97	97	61	61
PD-L1 (TCs)	Correlation coefficient	−0.110	−0.171	1.000	0.383 **	0.242	0.175
	Sig. (2-tailed) *	0.283	0.094	-	0.000	0.060	0.177
	No.	97	97	97	97	61	61
PD-L1 (ICs)	Correlation coefficient	−0.155	−0.259 *	0.383 **	1.000	0.429 **	0.470 **
	Sig. (2-tailed) *	0.129	0.010	0.000	-	0.001	0.000
	No.	97	97	97	97	61	61
CD43 (ICs)	Correlation coefficient	−0.091	−0.247	0.242	0.429 **	1.000	0.608 **
	Sig. (2-tailed) *	0.485	0.055	0.060	0.001	-	0.000
	No.	61	61	61	61	61	61
CD8 (ICs)	Correlation coefficient	−0.021	−0.126	0.175	0.470 **	0.608 **	1.000
	Sig. (2-tailed) *	0.875	0.334	0.177	0.000	0.000	-
	No.	61	61	61	61	61	61

**, Correlation is significant at the 0.01 level (2-tailed); *, Correlation is significant at the 0.05 level (2-tailed); TC, tumor cell; IC, immune cell.

It has been observed that expression of CD43 and CD8 in tumor microenvironment ICs is generally predominant in the lamina propria rather than the muscle layer. Since CD8 and CD43 expression showed various degrees according to the depth of tumor infiltration, intra-tumoral or contiguous peritumoral ICs in the muscularis propria and deeper layer were evaluated in 61 cases of pT2–pT4 (Figure 2).

3.4. Expression of HER2 or IDO May Predict Shorter Disease-Free Survival Period in 69 Cases of pT2–pT4

In pT2–pT4 cases ($n = 69$), we found that expression of HER2 or IDO in TCs was associated with a shorter DFS in both univariate Cox regression analysis ($p = 0.028$ and $p = 0.048$, respectively) (Table 3) and Kaplan–Meier survival curves ($p = 0.022$ and $p = 0.040$, respectively) (Figure 3). The expression of HER2 in TCs was also associated with shorter OS and DFS periods according to multivariate Cox regression analysis for HER2 expression, IDO expression, gender, age, pathologic tumor stage, and radiation therapy after surgery ($p = 0.031$ and $p = 0.019$, respectively) (Table 4). The PD-L1 expression in TCs or ICs showed no correlation with survival outcome (Table 3 and Figure 3), even though the PD-L1 expression of ICs was higher in pT2–pT4 than in pTa–pT1 ($p = 0.001$). The expression of CD43 and CD8 in ICs showed no correlation with survival outcome. In 29 cases of pT2–pT4 with radiation therapy after surgery, the expression of HER2 or IDO in TCs showed an association with shorter DFS in Kaplan–Meier survival curves ($p = 0.061$ and $p = 0.033$) (Figure 4).

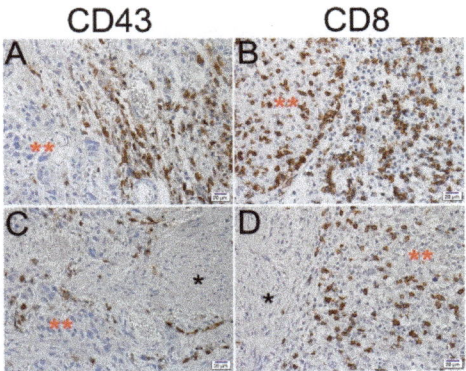

Figure 2. Representative images of CD43 and CD8 immunohistochemical staining in urothelial carcinoma of the bladder (UCB). Positive expression of CD43 and CD8 in intra-tumoral or contiguous peritumoral immune cells of lamina propria invasion (**A**,**B**) and muscularis propria (**C**,**D**) (scale bar = 20 μm; *, muscularis propria; and **, tumor cells).

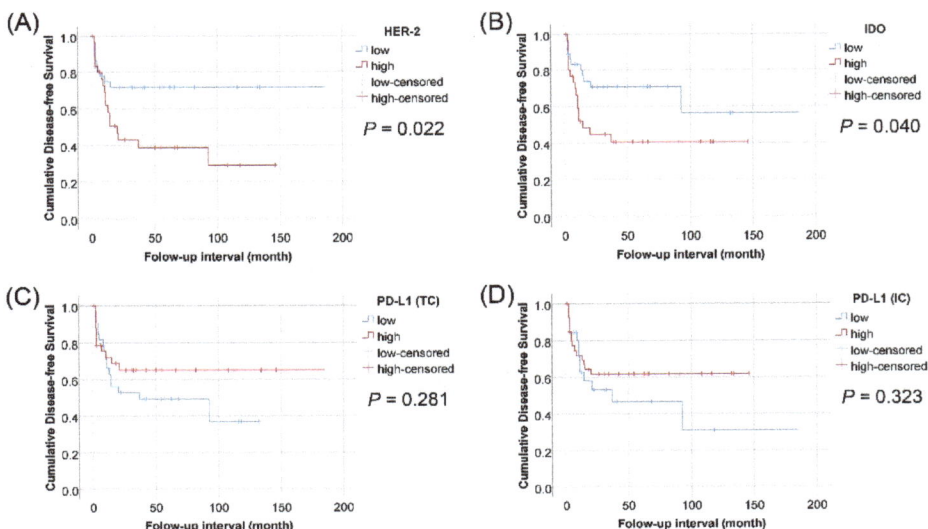

Figure 3. Kaplan–Meier survival curves of disease-free survival in 69 patients with pathologic tumor stage pT2–pT4 urothelial carcinoma of the bladder according to expression of HER2 in tumor cells, IDO in tumor cells, PD-L1 in tumor cells, and PD-L1 in immune cells. (**A**) HER2; (**B**) IDO; (**C**) PD-L1 (TCs); (**D**) PD-L1 (ICs)).

Table 3. Univariate analysis of overall survival and disease-free survival in 69 patients with pathologic tumor stage pT2–pT4 urothelial carcinoma of the bladder.

	Overall Survival			Disease-free Survival		
	P *	HR	95% CI	P *	HR	95% CI
HER2 expression (TCs)	0.143			0.028		
Low		1 (reference)			1 (reference)	
High		1.792	0.822–3.907		2.381	1.097–5.169
IDO expression (TCs)	0.683			0.048		
Low		1 (reference)			1 (reference)	
High		0.850	0.390–1.852		2.158	1.007–4.622
PD-L1 expression (TCs)	0.854			0.291		
Low		1 (reference)			1 (reference)	
High		1.075	0.498–2.320		0.664	0.311–1.420
PD-L1 expression (ICs)	0.741			0.333		
Low		1 (reference)			1 (reference)	
High		1.146	0.510–2.577		0.692	0.329–1.458
Gender	0.360			0.164		
Male		1 (reference)			1 (reference)	
Female		0.605	0.206–1.774		0.425	0.128–1.417
Age (years)	0.357			0.922		
≤65		1 (reference)			1 (reference)	
>65		1.481	0.643–3.413		0.962	0.444–2.085
Tumor stage	0.016			0.804		
pT2		1 (reference)			1 (reference)	
pT3–pT4		2.639	1.196–5.824		1.100	0.520–2.326
Radiation therapy after surgery	0.395			0.716		
No		1 (reference)			1 (reference)	
Yes		0.706	0.316–1.576		0.870	0.410–1.844

* univariate Cox regression analysis; HR, hazard ratio; CI, confidence interval; TC, tumor cell; IC, immune cell.

Table 4. Multivariate analysis of overall survival and disease-free survival in 69 patients with pathologic tumor stage pT2–pT4 urothelial carcinoma of the bladder.

	Overall Survival			Disease-free Survival		
	P	HR	95% CI	P	HR	95% CI
HER2 expression (TCs)	0.031			0.019		
Low		1 (reference)			1 (reference)	
High		2.501	1.090–5.743		2.729	0.076–6.332
IDO expression (TCs)	0.545			0.101		
Low		1 (reference)			1 (reference)	
High		0.772	0.334–1.786		1.988	0.876–4.514
Gender	0.350			0.054		
Male		1 (reference)			1 (reference)	
Female		0.576	0.181–1.833		0.283	0.078–1.024

Table 4. Cont.

		Overall Survival			Disease-free Survival	
	P	HR	95% CI	P	HR	95% CI
Age (years)	0.107			0.858		
≤65		1 (reference)			1 (reference)	
>65		2.036	0.858–4.833		1.079	0.470–2.475
Tumor stage	0.045			0.886		
pT2		1 (reference)			1 (reference)	
pT3–pT4		2.424	1.020–5.760		0.942	0.419–2.113
Radiation therapy after surgery	0.744			0.505		
No		1 (reference)			1 (reference)	
Yes		0.867	0.369–2.039		0.766	0.350–1.675

* multivariate Cox regression analysis; HR, hazard ratio; CI, confidence interval; TC, tumor cell; IC, immune cell.

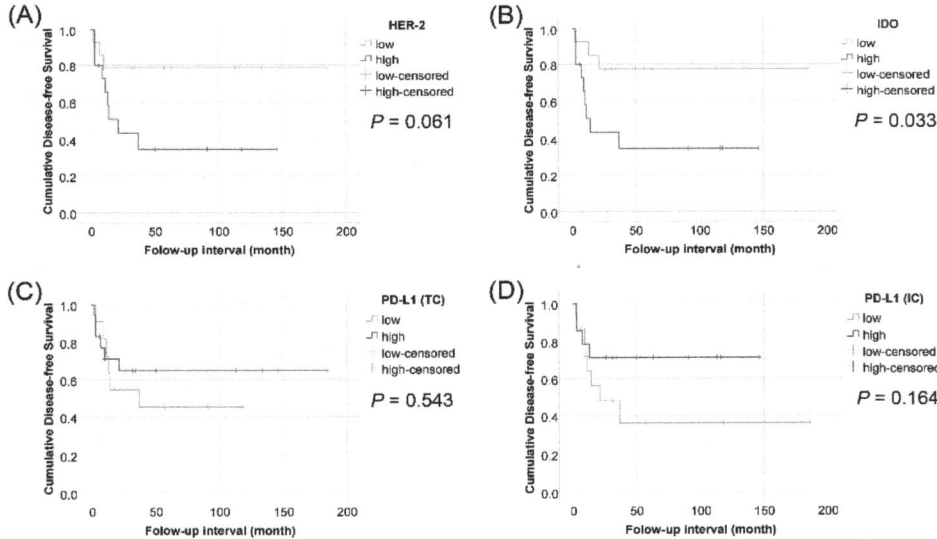

Figure 4. Kaplan–Meier survival curves of disease-free survival in 29 cases with post-operative radiotherapy among 69 patients of pathologic tumor stage pT2–pT4 urothelial carcinoma of the bladder, according to expression of HER2 in tumor cells, IDO in tumor cells, PD-L1 in tumor cells, and PD-L1 in immune cells. (**A**) HER2; (**B**) IDO; (**C**) PD-L1 (TCs); (**D**) PD-L1 (ICs)).

4. Discussion

In this study, we evaluated the expression of HER2, IDO, and PD-L1 in 97 UCB cases. The three proteins showed a correlation with tumor progression or patient outcome, although they did not show the same trends for clinicopathological correlations. We demonstrated that PD-L1 expression in ICs was significantly higher in pT2–pT4 than in pTa–pT1. Increased HER2 and IDO levels in TCs of 69 pT2–pT4 cases were positively correlated with a shorter DFS period, and could be considered potential factors in poor disease outcomes.

The roles of HER2 and IDO protein in cancer initiation or progression are still poorly understood. The consistent association between the effects of anti-HER2 therapies and immune infiltration has been reported in breast cancer and supports that an anti-tumor immune response can modulate the effect of anti-HER2 therapy [30,31]. In our study, the invasive UCB cancer cells showed a relatively reduced expression of HER2 or IDO in comparison to the expression of reactive or dysplastic intraepithelial urothelial cells. In pTa–pT1 UCBs, the expression of HER2 and IDO increased relative to that of pT2–pT4, apart from that, in pT2–pT4 cases, increased expressions of the two proteins are associated with reduced DFS expression. The altered expression of IDO or HER2 could be interpreted to be a different phase or play a different role for cancer immunoediting to the immune response against noninvasive UCB and invasive UCB [30,32,33]. Our data show a significant positive correlation between the expression of PD-L1, CD43 and CD8 in ICs. It has been observed that there is higher expression of CD43 and CD8 in lamina propria invasion in comparison to muscularis propria invasion. Moreover, there was a tendency to have a reverse correlation between the expression of IDO and HER2 in TCs and the expression of PD-L1, CD43 and CD8 in ICs. Cancer immunoediting describes a complex mechanism between ICs and TCs and has three phases: elimination, equilibrium and escape [34]. In the final escape phase, the expression of IDO in cancer cells inhibits the host immune protection. Paradoxically, IDO is elevated upon various immune molecules of adaptive or innate or tolerogenic immune cells. We speculate that elevated levels of IDO and HER2 in TC may reflect a tumor microenvironment immune reaction. And those immune-evasive transformed cancer cells may reduce IDO expression after down-regulation of immune response with a negative feedback mechanism [30,33,35]. It is predicted that in early cancer development, the expression of IDO or HER2 is upregulated in the majority of cancer cells stimulated by various immune molecules, including IFN-γ, IL-10, IL-27, CTLA4, TGF-β, cyclooxygenase-2 and prostaglandin E2, which are regulated by tumor antigen level or tolerogenic tumor microenvironment [33]. In advanced invasive cancer, the two proteins could be continuously expressed in a relatively reduced number of poorly immunogenic and immune evasive transformed cancer cells, which can lead to a poor prognosis [34]. Therefore, a spatial and periodic variety of cancer immunoediting phase could be in the same tumor mass.

In UCB, HER2 expression status has been evaluated since 1990, when overexpression of HER2 protein was first reported [36]. One study of high-grade UCB (pT2–pT4) ranked the *HER2* gene amplification as the third most significant in terms of associated genetic mutations [37]. Although the first study on the relationship of HER2 expression with clinical outcomes is confounding, a meta-analysis has indicated that its expression is associated with tumor grade, lymph node metastasis, and poor prognosis in UCB [38]. Even so, recent studies have not produced encouraging results for HER2 targeted therapy as a strategy against UCB [39–41]. The major scientific reasons for the failure of HER2 targeted therapy are a lack of standardization of HER2 testing and co-expression of other immunomodulatory molecules [42]. To overcome the poor results achieved thus far with anti-HER2 therapy, it is necessary to identify correlations between HER2 and immune checkpoint proteins in UCB. Our study reported that HER2 expression is marginally associated with IDO expression. To the best of our knowledge, this is the first study to correlate HER2 and immunosuppressive molecules in UCB.

Anti-HER2 therapy has revolutionized the treatment of malignant tumors, especially overexpressing breast cancer. Furthermore, with increasing concentrations of anticancer immunotherapy, the connection between HER2 expression and antitumor immunity has emerged as a possible target for combined oncological treatment. The whole-transcriptome profiling of HER2-positive breast carcinomas has revealed a remarkable enrichment in immune pathways [43]. HER2-positive trastuzumab-sensitive breast carcinomas have shown positive associations with chemokines involved in immune cell infiltration of the tumor microenvironment and the expression of PD-1 ligands in tumor cells [16,44]. HER2 expression has recently been found to suppress antiviral defenses and antitumor immunity as a result of HER2 signaling through its intracellular domain, which interferes with cyclic GMP-AMP synthase-stimulator of interferon genes (cGAS-STING) pathway and prevents cancer cell death [45]. Therefore, innate and adaptive immune system responses are increasingly being acknowledged as important regulators of the effects of HER2 targeted therapy [46,47]. Based on previous research, in this study HER2 expression was scored in the cytoplasm as well as the cytoplasmic membrane to include the immune systemic function of the intracellular domain of HER2 signaling. Considering the role of HER2 protein in interfering with antitumor immunity in the cytoplasm, the indications for HER2 targeted therapy are not limited to the cytoplasmic membrane expression of HER2 and we expect that they may also be extended to HER2 protein expression in the cytoplasm of cancer cells.

IDO, also referred to as IDO1, is one of the cytosolic enzymes that catalyzes the initial and rate-limiting steps of tryptophan to kynurenine [33,48]. IDO has been described as having immunosuppressive functions on host immune surveillance of tumor cells, with a focus on its potential immunotherapeutic targets [49]. The role of IDO has been implicated in immune tolerance related to the suppression of T-cell responses such as fetal tolerance, tumor resistance, chronic infections, and autoimmune diseases [50]. One study delineated the action of kynurenine to promote apoptosis in murine bone marrow-derived neutrophils, providing a possible mechanism for increased neutrophil accumulation in IDO-deficient mice [51]. Our results show that IDO expression is correlated with increased ALC and decreased ANC. These findings support previous studies on the immunomodulatory functions of IDO, although its effects or mechanisms in tumor progression remain unclear. IDO expression in TCs showed a negative correlation with ANC and positive correlation with ALC, while the PD-L1 expression in ICs was positively correlated with ANC in the 97 UCB cases.

Recently, phase II and preliminary phase III studies have shown that the application of a PD-L1 inhibitor in metastatic platinum-refractory NSCLC and urothelial cancer resulted in a significant improvement in the response rate and median overall survival [52]. Furthermore, PD-L1 tumor expression has emerged as a biomarker for patient stratification in immunotherapy targeting for the PD-L1/PD-1 pathway, particularly for NSCLC [53]. However, the prognostic impact of this molecule in tumor tissue is still controversial in various cancers, such as NSCLC and head and neck squamous cell carcinoma, because of the high discrepancies between PD-L1 expression and treatment outcomes [54,55]. Some studies have emphasized the significance of a comprehensive evaluation of PD-L1 expression on tumor and immune cells because its expression in immune cells, but not tumor cells, is a favorable prognostic factor for NSCLC and HNSCC [55–57]. However, our results show that PD-L1 expression in ICs is a significant poor prognostic factor in UCB.

Radiotherapy induces a host immune response by exposing tumor-specific antigens that make tumor cells detectable by the immune system, promoting the priming and activation of cytotoxic T cells [58]. Furthermore, radiation may have an impact on the tumor microenvironment by facilitating the recruitment and infiltration of immune cells [58–60]. Although radiotherapy acts as an in-situ tumor vaccine, it may be insufficient to sustain long-term antitumor immunity, resulting in later relapse [61]. Therefore, there are many studies identifying correlations between molecular regulators of tumor immune escapes and radio-resistance. PD-L1 positive cancer cells have been demonstrated to have a radio-resistant phenotype, inhibiting T cell signaling and T cell-mediated immunogenic cell death [62]. HER2 activation is a potential mechanism that may compromise the outcome of radiotherapy [63,64]. Additionally, in vitro and in vivo experiments blocking PD-L1 and IDO alongside radiation have successfully overcome rebound immune suppression [65,66]. Similarly, our data reveal that the expression of HER2 and IDO are significantly associated with DFS in UCB treated with radiotherapy after surgery (Figure 4).

5. Conclusions

The present study is the first to measure the expression levels of IDO, HER2, and PD-L1 and to analyze the correlation between these three proteins and clinicopathological values in UCB. The expression of IDO and HER2 in TCs and PD-L1 in ICs were positively correlated with poor prognostic factors in pT2–pT4 cases, including shorter DFS and OS periods or higher tumor stage. Our results suggest that the expression of IDO, HER2, and PD-L1 are useful as predictive prognostic factors and could potentially be utilized for the development of combined cancer immunotherapeutic strategies.

Supplementary Materials: The following are available online at http://www.mdpi.com/2077-0383/9/5/1265/s1, Table S1: Candidate genes associated with CD8+ T cell infiltration in urothelial carcinoma of the bladder., Table S2:

Correlations of HER2, IDO, and PD-L1 expressions with hematologic parameters in 97 patients with urothelial carcinoma of the bladder, Figure S1: Kaplan-Meier survival curves comparing the high and low infiltrating levels of CD8+ T cells, CD4+ T cells, macrophages, neutrophils, and dendritic cells in urothelial carcinoma of the bladder.

Author Contributions: Conceptualization, K.-H.K.; Data curation, K.-H.K., D.K. and S.K.; Funding acquisition, K.-H.K. and S.K.; Investigation, K.-H.K., D.K. and S.K.; Methodology, S.K. and K.-H.K.; Project administration, K.-H.K.; Resources, J.-S.K., J.M.K., S.K. and K.-H.K.; Supervision, K.-H.K.; Validation, S.K. and J.M.K.; Writing–original draft, S.K. and K.-H.K.; Writing–review & editing, D.K., J.M.K., J.-S.K., S.K. and K.-H.K. All authors have read and agreed to the published version of the manuscript.

Funding: This work was supported by the Basic Science Research Program through the National Research Foundation of Korea (NRF), funded by the Ministry of Education, Science, and Technology (NRF-2016R1D1A1B01014311; K.-H. K. and NRF-2019M3E5D1A02068546; S. K.).

Conflicts of Interest: The authors declare no conflicts of interest. The funders had no role in the design of the study; the collection, analyses, or interpretation of data; the writing of the manuscript, or in the decision to publish these results.

References

1. Siegel, R.; Naishadham, D.; Jemal, A. Cancer statistics, 2012. *CA Cancer J. Clin.* **2012**, *62*, 10–29. [CrossRef] [PubMed]
2. Kirkali, Z.; Chan, T.; Manoharan, M.; Algaba, F.; Busch, C.; Cheng, L.; Kiemeney, L.; Kriegmair, M.; Montironi, R.; Murphy, W.M.; et al. Bladder cancer: Epidemiology, staging and grading, and diagnosis. *Urology* **2005**, *66*, 4–34. [CrossRef] [PubMed]
3. Porter, M.P.; Kerrigan, M.C.; Donato, B.M.; Ramsey, S.D. Patterns of use of systemic chemotherapy for Medicare beneficiaries with urothelial bladder cancer. *Urol. Oncol.* **2011**, *29*, 252–258. [CrossRef] [PubMed]
4. Meeks, J.J.; Bellmunt, J.; Bochner, B.H.; Clarke, N.W.; Daneshmand, S.; Galsky, M.D.; Hahn, N.M.; Lerner, S.P.; Mason, M.; Powles, T.; et al. A systematic review of neoadjuvant and adjuvant chemotherapy for muscle-invasive bladder cancer. *Eur. Urol.* **2012**, *62*, 523–533. [CrossRef] [PubMed]
5. Helmy, K.Y.; Patel, S.A.; Nahas, G.R.; Rameshwar, P. Cancer immunotherapy: Accomplishments to date and future promise. *Ther. Deliv.* **2013**, *4*, 1307–1320. [CrossRef] [PubMed]
6. Salmon, H.; Remark, R.; Gnjatic, S.; Merad, M. Host tissue determinants of tumour immunity. *Nat. Rev. Cancer* **2019**, *19*, 215–227. [CrossRef]
7. Box, C.; Rogers, S.J.; Mendiola, M.; Eccles, S.A. Tumour-microenvironmental interactions: Paths to progression and targets for treatment. *Semin. Cancer Biol.* **2010**, *20*, 128–138. [CrossRef]
8. Blankenstein, T.; Coulie, P.G.; Gilboa, E.; Jaffee, E.M. The determinants of tumour immunogenicity. *Nat. Rev. Cancer* **2012**, *12*, 307–313. [CrossRef]
9. Kroemer, G.; Galluzzi, L.; Kepp, O.; Zitvogel, L. Immunogenic cell death in cancer therapy. *Annu. Rev. Immunol.* **2013**, *31*, 51–72. [CrossRef] [PubMed]
10. Krysko, D.V.; Garg, A.D.; Kaczmarek, A.; Krysko, O.; Agostinis, P.; Vandenabeele, P. Immunogenic cell death and DAMPs in cancer therapy. *Nat. Rev. Cancer* **2012**, *12*, 860–875. [CrossRef]
11. Huang, Y.; Zhang, S.D.; McCrudden, C.; Chan, K.W.; Lin, Y.; Kwok, H.F. The prognostic significance of PD-L1 in bladder cancer. *Oncol. Rep.* **2015**, *33*, 3075–3084. [CrossRef] [PubMed]
12. Hudolin, T.; Mengus, C.; Coulot, J.; Kastelan, Z.; El-Saleh, A.; Spagnoli, G.C. Expression of Indoleamine 2,3-Dioxygenase Gene Is a Feature of Poorly Differentiated Non-muscle-invasive Urothelial Cell Bladder Carcinomas. *Anticancer Res.* **2017**, *37*, 1375–1380. [CrossRef] [PubMed]
13. Yang, C.; Zhou, Y.; Zhang, L.; Jin, C.; Li, M.; Ye, L. Expression and function analysis of indoleamine 2 and 3-dioxygenase in bladder urothelial carcinoma. *Int. J. Clin. Exp. Pathol.* **2015**, *8*, 1768–1775. [PubMed]
14. Chism, D.D. Urothelial Carcinoma of the Bladder and the Rise of Immunotherapy. *J. Natl. Compr. Canc. Netw.* **2017**, *15*, 1277–1284. [CrossRef]
15. Bellati, F.; Napoletano, C.; Ruscito, I.; Liberati, M.; Panici, P.B.; Nuti, M. Cellular adaptive immune system plays a crucial role in trastuzumab clinical efficacy. *J. Clin. Oncol.* **2010**, *28*, e369–e370. [CrossRef]
16. Triulzi, T.; Forte, L.; Regondi, V.; Di Modica, M.; Ghirelli, C.; Carcangiu, M.L.; Sfondrini, L.; Balsari, A.; Tagliabue, E. HER2 signaling regulates the tumor immune microenvironment and trastuzumab efficacy. *Oncoimmunology* **2019**, *8*, e1512942. [CrossRef]

17. Suh, K.J.; Sung, J.H.; Kim, J.W.; Han, S.H.; Lee, H.S.; Min, A.; Kang, M.H.; Kim, J.E.; Kim, J.W.; Kim, S.H.; et al. EGFR or HER2 inhibition modulates the tumor microenvironment by suppression of PD-L1 and cytokines release. *Oncotarget* **2017**, *8*, 63901–63910. [CrossRef]
18. Soliman, H.; Rawal, B.; Fulp, J.; Lee, J.H.; Lopez, A.; Bui, M.M.; Khalil, F.; Antonia, S.; Yfantis, H.G.; Lee, D.H.; et al. Analysis of indoleamine 2-3 dioxygenase (IDO1) expression in breast cancer tissue by immunohistochemistry. *Cancer Immunol. Immunother.* **2013**, *62*, 829–837. [CrossRef]
19. Amin, M.; Edge, S.; Greene, F.; Byrd, D.R.; Brookland, R.K.; Washington, M.K. *AJCC Cancer Staging Manual*, 8th ed.; Springer: Chicago, IL, USA, 2017.
20. Yeo, M.K.; Kim, J.M.; Suh, K.S.; Kim, S.H.; Lee, O.J.; Kim, K.H. Decreased Expression of the Polarity Regulatory PAR Complex Predicts Poor Prognosis of the Patients with Colorectal Adenocarcinoma. *Transl. Oncol.* **2018**, *11*, 109–115. [CrossRef]
21. HercepTest™, Interpretation Manual Breast Cancer. Available online: https://www.agilent.com/cs/library/usermanuals/public/28630_herceptest_interpretation_manual-breast_ihc_row.pdf (accessed on 26 April 2020).
22. PD-L1 IHC 22C3 pharmDx Interpretation Manual—Urothelial Carcinoma. Available online: https://www.agilent.com/cs/library/usermanuals/public/29276_22C3_pharmdx_uc_interpretation_manual_us.pdf (accessed on 26 April 2020).
23. VENTANA PD-L1 (SP142) Assay. Available online: https://www.accessdata.fda.gov/cdrh_docs/pdf16/P160002c.pdf (accessed on 26 April 2020).
24. Allred, D.C.; Harvey, J.M.; Berardo, M.; Clark, G.M. Prognostic and predictive factors in breast cancer by immunohistochemical analysis. *Mod. Pathol.* **1998**, *11*, 155–168.
25. Li, T.; Fan, J.; Wang, B.; Traugh, N.; Chen, Q.; Liu, J.S.; Li, B.; Liu, X.S. TIMER: A Web Server for Comprehensive Analysis of Tumor-Infiltrating Immune Cells. *Cancer Res.* **2017**, *77*, e108–e110. [CrossRef] [PubMed]
26. Li, B.; Severson, E.; Pignon, J.C.; Zhao, H.; Li, T.; Novak, J.; Jiang, P.; Shen, H.; Aster, J.C.; Rodig, S.; et al. Comprehensive analyses of tumor immunity: Implications for cancer immunotherapy. *Genome Biol.* **2016**, *17*, 174. [CrossRef]
27. Rabinovich, G.A.; Gabrilovich, D.; Sotomayor, E.M. Immunosuppressive strategies that are mediated by tumor cells. *Annu. Rev. Immunol.* **2007**, *25*, 267–296. [CrossRef] [PubMed]
28. Crispen, P.L.; Kusmartsev, S. Mechanisms of immune evasion in bladder cancer. *Cancer Immunol. Immunother.* **2020**, *69*, 3–14. [CrossRef] [PubMed]
29. Liu, M.; Wang, X.; Wang, L.; Ma, X.; Gong, Z.; Zhang, S.; Li, Y. Targeting the IDO1 pathway in cancer: From bench to bedside. *J. Hematol. Oncol.* **2018**, *11*, 100. [CrossRef] [PubMed]
30. Teng, M.W.; Galon, J.; Fridman, W.H.; Smyth, M.J. From mice to humans: Developments in cancer immunoediting. *J. Clin. Investig.* **2015**, *125*, 3338–3346. [CrossRef] [PubMed]
31. Bianchini, G.; Gianni, L. The immune system and response to HER2-targeted treatment in breast cancer. *Lancet Oncol.* **2014**, *15*, e58–e68. [CrossRef]
32. Kim, R.; Emi, M.; Tanabe, K. Cancer immunoediting from immune surveillance to immune escape. *Immunology* **2007**, *121*, 1–14. [CrossRef]
33. Hornyak, L.; Dobos, N.; Koncz, G.; Karanyi, Z.; Pall, D.; Szabo, Z.; Halmos, G.; Szekvolgyi, L. The Role of Indoleamine-2,3-Dioxygenase in Cancer Development, Diagnostics, and Therapy. *Front. Immunol.* **2018**, *9*, 151. [CrossRef]
34. Schreiber, R.D.; Old, L.J.; Smyth, M.J. Cancer immunoediting: Integrating immunity's roles in cancer suppression and promotion. *Science* **2011**, *331*, 1565–1570. [CrossRef]
35. Spranger, S.; Spaapen, R.M.; Zha, Y.; Williams, J.; Meng, Y.; Ha, T.T.; Gajewski, T.F. Up-regulation of PD-L1, IDO, and T(regs) in the melanoma tumor microenvironment is driven by CD8(+) T cells. *Sci. Transl. Med.* **2013**, *5*, 200ra116. [CrossRef]
36. Wright, C.; Mellon, K.; Neal, D.E.; Johnston, P.; Corbett, I.P.; Horne, C.H. Expression of c-erbB-2 protein product in bladder cancer. *Br. J. Cancer* **1990**, *62*, 764–765. [CrossRef] [PubMed]
37. Cancer Genome Atlas Research Network. Comprehensive molecular characterization of urothelial bladder carcinoma. *Nature* **2014**, *507*, 315–322. [CrossRef] [PubMed]
38. Zhao, J.; Xu, W.; Zhang, Z.; Song, R.; Zeng, S.; Sun, Y.; Xu, C. Prognostic role of HER2 expression in bladder cancer: A systematic review and meta-analysis. *Int. Urol. Nephrol.* **2015**, *47*, 87–94. [CrossRef] [PubMed]

39. Oudard, S.; Culine, S.; Vano, Y.; Goldwasser, F.; Theodore, C.; Nguyen, T.; Voog, E.; Banu, E.; Vieillefond, A.; Priou, F.; et al. Multicentre randomised phase II trial of gemcitabine+platinum, with or without trastuzumab, in advanced or metastatic urothelial carcinoma overexpressing Her2. *Eur. J. Cancer* **2015**, *51*, 45–54. [CrossRef] [PubMed]
40. Wulfing, C.; Machiels, J.P.; Richel, D.J.; Grimm, M.O.; Treiber, U.; De Groot, M.R.; Beuzeboc, P.; Parikh, R.; Petavy, F.; El-Hariry, I.A. A single-arm, multicenter, open-label phase 2 study of lapatinib as the second-line treatment of patients with locally advanced or metastatic transitional cell carcinoma. *Cancer* **2009**, *115*, 2881–2890. [CrossRef]
41. Powles, T.; Huddart, R.A.; Elliott, T.; Sarker, S.J.; Ackerman, C.; Jones, R.; Hussain, S.; Crabb, S.; Jagdev, S.; Chester, J.; et al. Phase III, Double-Blind, Randomized Trial That Compared Maintenance Lapatinib Versus Placebo After First-Line Chemotherapy in Patients with Human Epidermal Growth Factor Receptor 1/2-Positive Metastatic Bladder Cancer. *J. Clin. Oncol.* **2017**, *35*, 48–55. [CrossRef]
42. Koshkin, V.S.; O'Donnell, P.; Yu, E.Y.; Grivas, P. Systematic Review: Targeting HER2 in Bladder Cancer. *Bladder Cancer* **2019**, *5*, 1–12. [CrossRef]
43. Triulzi, T.; De Cecco, L.; Sandri, M.; Prat, A.; Giussani, M.; Paolini, B.; Carcangiu, M.L.; Canevari, S.; Bottini, A.; Balsari, A.; et al. Whole-transcriptome analysis links trastuzumab sensitivity of breast tumors to both HER2 dependence and immune cell infiltration. *Oncotarget* **2015**, *6*, 28173–28182. [CrossRef]
44. Gil Del Alcazar, C.R.; Huh, S.J.; Ekram, M.B.; Trinh, A.; Liu, L.L.; Beca, F.; Zi, X.; Kwak, M.; Bergholtz, H.; Su, Y.; et al. Immune Escape in Breast Cancer During In Situ to Invasive Carcinoma Transition. *Cancer Discov.* **2017**, *7*, 1098–1115. [CrossRef]
45. Wu, S.; Zhang, Q.; Zhang, F.; Meng, F.; Liu, S.; Zhou, R.; Wu, Q.; Li, X.; Shen, L.; Huang, J.; et al. HER2 recruits AKT1 to disrupt STING signalling and suppress antiviral defence and antitumour immunity. *Nat. Cell Biol.* **2019**, *21*, 1027–1040. [CrossRef]
46. Verma, S.; Miles, D.; Gianni, L.; Krop, I.E.; Welslau, M.; Baselga, J.; Pegram, M.; Oh, D.Y.; Dieras, V.; Guardino, E.; et al. Trastuzumab emtansine for HER2-positive advanced breast cancer. *N. Engl. J. Med.* **2012**, *367*, 1783–1791. [CrossRef] [PubMed]
47. Ferris, R.L.; Jaffee, E.M.; Ferrone, S. Tumor antigen-targeted, monoclonal antibody-based immunotherapy: Clinical response, cellular immunity, and immunoescape. *J. Clin. Oncol.* **2010**, *28*, 4390–4399. [CrossRef] [PubMed]
48. Brochez, L.; Chevolet, I.; Kruse, V. The rationale of indoleamine 2,3-dioxygenase inhibition for cancer therapy. *Eur. J. Cancer* **2017**, *76*, 167–182. [CrossRef] [PubMed]
49. Zhu, M.M.T.; Dancsok, A.R.; Nielsen, T.O. Indoleamine Dioxygenase Inhibitors: Clinical Rationale and Current Development. *Curr. Oncol. Rep.* **2019**, *21*, 2. [CrossRef]
50. Mellor, A.L.; Munn, D.H. IDO expression by dendritic cells: Tolerance and tryptophan catabolism. *Nat. Rev. Immunol.* **2004**, *4*, 762–774. [CrossRef]
51. El-Zaatari, M.; Chang, Y.M.; Zhang, M.; Franz, M.; Shreiner, A.; McDermott, A.J.; van der Sluijs, K.F.; Lutter, R.; Grasberger, H.; Kamada, N.; et al. Tryptophan catabolism restricts IFN-gamma-expressing neutrophils and Clostridium difficile immunopathology. *J. Immunol.* **2014**, *193*, 807–816. [CrossRef]
52. Krishnamurthy, A.; Jimeno, A. Atezolizumab: A novel PD-L1 inhibitor in cancer therapy with a focus in bladder and non-small cell lung cancers. *Drugs Today* **2017**, *53*, 217–237. [CrossRef]
53. Brody, R.; Zhang, Y.; Ballas, M.; Siddiqui, M.K.; Gupta, P.; Barker, C.; Midha, A.; Walker, J. PD-L1 expression in advanced NSCLC: Insights into risk stratification and treatment selection from a systematic literature review. *Lung Cancer* **2017**, *112*, 200–215. [CrossRef]
54. Takada, K.; Okamoto, T.; Toyokawa, G.; Kozuma, Y.; Matsubara, T.; Haratake, N.; Akamine, T.; Takamori, S.; Katsura, M.; Shoji, F.; et al. The expression of PD-L1 protein as a prognostic factor in lung squamous cell carcinoma. *Lung Cancer* **2017**, *104*, 7–15. [CrossRef]
55. Kim, H.R.; Ha, S.J.; Hong, M.H.; Heo, S.J.; Koh, Y.W.; Choi, E.C.; Kim, E.K.; Pyo, K.H.; Jung, I.; Seo, D.; et al. PD-L1 expression on immune cells, but not on tumor cells, is a favorable prognostic factor for head and neck cancer patients. *Sci. Rep.* **2016**, *6*, 36956. [CrossRef] [PubMed]
56. Bocanegra, A.; Fernandez-Hinojal, G.; Zuazo-Ibarra, M.; Arasanz, H.; Garcia-Granda, M.J.; Hernandez, C.; Ibanez, M.; Hernandez-Marin, B.; Martinez-Aguillo, M.; Lecumberri, M.J.; et al. PD-L1 Expression in Systemic Immune Cell Populations as a Potential Predictive Biomarker of Responses to PD-L1/PD-1 Blockade Therapy in Lung Cancer. *Int. J. Mol. Sci.* **2019**, *20*, 1631. [CrossRef] [PubMed]

57. Birtalan, E.; Danos, K.; Gurbi, B.; Brauswetter, D.; Halasz, J.; Kalocsane Piurko, V.; Acs, B.; Antal, B.; Mihalyi, R.; Pato, A.; et al. Expression of PD-L1 on Immune Cells Shows Better Prognosis in Laryngeal, Oropharyngeal, and Hypopharyngeal Cancer. *Appl. Immunohistochem. Mol. Morphol.* **2018**, *26*, e79–e85. [CrossRef] [PubMed]
58. Formenti, S.C.; Demaria, S. Combining radiotherapy and cancer immunotherapy: A paradigm shift. *J. Natl. Cancer Inst.* **2013**, *105*, 256–265. [CrossRef] [PubMed]
59. McBride, W.H.; Chiang, C.S.; Olson, J.L.; Wang, C.C.; Hong, J.H.; Pajonk, F.; Dougherty, G.J.; Iwamoto, K.S.; Pervan, M.; Liao, Y.P. A sense of danger from radiation. *Radiat. Res.* **2004**, *162*, 1–19. [CrossRef]
60. Haikerwal, S.J.; Hagekyriakou, J.; MacManus, M.; Martin, O.A.; Haynes, N.M. Building immunity to cancer with radiation therapy. *Cancer Lett.* **2015**, *368*, 198–208. [CrossRef]
61. Wennerberg, E.; Lhuillier, C.; Vanpouille-Box, C.; Pilones, K.A.; Garcia-Martinez, E.; Rudqvist, N.P.; Formenti, S.C.; Demaria, S. Barriers to Radiation-Induced In Situ Tumor Vaccination. *Front. Immunol.* **2017**, *8*, 229. [CrossRef]
62. Lyu, X.; Zhang, M.; Li, G.; Jiang, Y.; Qiao, Q. PD-1 and PD-L1 Expression Predicts Radiosensitivity and Clinical Outcomes in Head and Neck Cancer and is Associated with HPV Infection. *J. Cancer* **2019**, *10*, 937–948. [CrossRef]
63. Duru, N.; Fan, M.; Candas, D.; Menaa, C.; Liu, H.C.; Nantajit, D.; Wen, Y.; Xiao, K.; Eldridge, A.; Chromy, B.A.; et al. HER2-associated radioresistance of breast cancer stem cells isolated from HER2-negative breast cancer cells. *Clin. Cancer Res.* **2012**, *18*, 6634–6647. [CrossRef]
64. Cao, N.; Li, S.; Wang, Z.; Ahmed, K.M.; Degnan, M.E.; Fan, M.; Dynlacht, J.R.; Li, J.J. NF-kappaB-mediated HER2 overexpression in radiation-adaptive resistance. *Radiat. Res.* **2009**, *171*, 9–21. [CrossRef]
65. Liu, M.; Li, Z.; Yao, W.; Zeng, X.; Wang, L.; Cheng, J.; Ma, B.; Zhang, R.; Min, W.; Wang, H. IDO inhibitor synergized with radiotherapy to delay tumor growth by reversing T cell exhaustion. *Mol. Med. Rep.* **2020**, *21*, 445–453. [CrossRef]
66. Ladomersky, E.; Zhai, L.; Lenzen, A.; Lauing, K.L.; Qian, J.; Scholtens, D.M.; Gritsina, G.; Sun, X.; Liu, Y.; Yu, F.; et al. IDO1 Inhibition Synergizes with Radiation and PD-1 Blockade to Durably Increase Survival Against Advanced Glioblastoma. *Clin. Cancer Res.* **2018**, *24*, 2559–2573. [CrossRef]

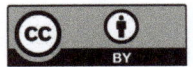

© 2020 by the authors. Licensee MDPI, Basel, Switzerland. This article is an open access article distributed under the terms and conditions of the Creative Commons Attribution (CC BY) license (http://creativecommons.org/licenses/by/4.0/).

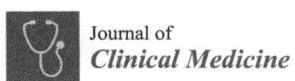

Article

FOXA1 Gene Expression for Defining Molecular Subtypes of Muscle-Invasive Bladder Cancer after Radical Cystectomy

Danijel Sikic [1,*], Markus Eckstein [2], Ralph M. Wirtz [3], Jonas Jarczyk [4], Thomas S. Worst [4], Stefan Porubsky [5], Bastian Keck [1], Frank Kunath [1], Veronika Weyerer [2], Johannes Breyer [6], Wolfgang Otto [6], Sebastien Rinaldetti [7], Christian Bolenz [8], Arndt Hartmann [2], Bernd Wullich [1] and Philipp Erben [4] on behalf of the BRIDGE Consortium e.V., Germany

[1] Department of Urology and Pediatric Urology, University Hospital Erlangen, Friedrich-Alexander University Erlangen-Nuremberg, 91054 Erlangen, Germany; bastian.keck@web.de (B.K.); frank.kunath@uk-erlangen.de (F.K.); bernd.wullich@uk-erlangen.de (B.W.)
[2] Institute of Pathology, University Hospital Erlangen, Friedrich-Alexander University Erlangen-Nuremberg, 91054 Erlangen, Germany; markus.eckstein@uk-erlangen.de (M.E.); veronika.weyerer@uk-erlangen.de (V.W.); arndt.hartmann@uk-erlangen.de (A.H.)
[3] STRATIFYER Molecular Pathology GmbH, 50935 Cologne, Germany; ralph.wirtz@STRATIFYER.de
[4] Department of Urology, University Medical Centre Mannheim, Medical Faculty Mannheim, University of Heidelberg, 68167 Mannheim, Germany; jonas.jarczyk@umm.de (J.J.); thomas.worst@umm.de (T.S.W.); philipp.erben@medma.uni-heidelberg.de (P.E.)
[5] Institute of Pathology, University Medical Centre Mannheim, Medical Faculty Mannheim, University of Heidelberg, 68167 Mannheim, Germany; stefan.porubsky@umm.de
[6] Department of Urology, University of Regensburg, 93053 Regensburg, Germany; johannes.breyer@ukr.de (J.B.); wolfgang.otto@ukr.de (W.O.)
[7] Department of Hematology and Oncology, University Medical Centre Mannheim, Medical Faculty Mannheim, University of Heidelberg, 68167 Mannheim, Germany; sebastien.rinaldetti@medma.uni-heidelberg.de
[8] Department of Urology and Pediatric Urology, University Hospital Ulm, 89081 Ulm, Germany; christian.bolenz@uniklinik-ulm.de
* Correspondence: danijel.sikic@uk-erlangen.de; Tel.: +49-9131-822-3178

Received: 4 March 2020; Accepted: 31 March 2020; Published: 2 April 2020

Abstract: It remains unclear how to implement the recently revealed basal and luminal subtypes of muscle-invasive bladder cancer (MIBC) into daily clinical routine and whether molecular marker panels can be reduced. The mRNA expression of basal (KRT5) and luminal (FOXA1, GATA3, KRT20) markers was measured by reverse transcription quantitative real-time polymerase chain reaction (RT-qPCR) and correlated to clinicopathological features, recurrence-free survival (RFS), disease-free survival (DFS), and overall survival (OS) in 80 patients with MIBC who underwent radical cystectomy. Additionally, the correlation of single markers with the basal and non-basal subtypes defined by a 36-gene panel was examined and then validated in the TCGA (The Cancer Genome Atlas) cohort. High expression of FOXA1 ($p = 0.0048$) and KRT20 ($p = 0.0317$) was associated with reduced RFS. In the multivariable analysis, only FOXA1 remained an independent prognostic marker for DFS ($p = 0.0333$) and RFS ($p = 0.0310$). FOXA1 expression (AUC = 0.79; $p = 0.0007$) was closest to the combined marker expression (AUC = 0.79; $p = 0.0015$) in resembling the non-basal subtype defined by the 36-gene panel. FOXA1 in combination with KRT5 may be used to distinguish the basal and non-basal subtypes of MIBC.

Keywords: FOXA1; GATA3; KRT20; molecular markers; mRNA; muscle-invasive bladder cancer; PCR; urothelial carcinoma

1. Introduction

Urothelial carcinoma of the bladder (UCB) is the 10th most common cancer worldwide, with an estimated 549,000 new cases and 200,000 deaths per year [1]. While the majority of patients have non-muscle-invasive bladder cancer (NMIBC), approximately 25% of patients with UCB have muscle-invasive bladder cancer (MIBC) or metastases at the time of diagnosis [2]. While radical cystectomy and platin-based chemotherapy have remained the therapeutic standard for MIBC and metastatic disease in the last few decades, the treatment and follow-up of MIBC continues to be very challenging [3,4]. Radical cystectomy is associated with high rates of perioperative morbidity and mortality [5], and approximately 50% of patients experience distant disease recurrence after cystectomy, mostly within the first two years, although later recurrences have also been reported [6–8]. The median survival of patients treated with cisplatin-based chemotherapy for metastatic disease ranges between nine and 26 months [3]. The need for lifelong surveillance as well as high treatment costs result in UCB being the most expensive cancer per patient from diagnosis to death in the US [9–11]. Given the high costs and poor outcome of patients with UCB, there is a high demand for novel molecular markers to improve diagnostics and serve as targets for new therapies.

In recent years, several independent groups have demonstrated the existence of distinct molecular subtypes in UCB comparable to the molecular subtypes in breast cancer [12–16]. It was also shown that these molecular subtypes were associated with different outcomes and responses to chemotherapy [15,17]. While these findings bear great potential to improve the diagnostics and treatment of UCB in the future, there are still many uncertainties. Based on genetic expression patterns, most groups defined the basal and luminal subtypes of UCB by measuring the expression of hundreds of genes, which is not conveyable into daily clinical practice because of the high cost and effort [12–16]. The identification of relevant surrogate markers is necessary for the easy and feasible implementation of the molecular subtyping of UCB into daily clinical routine, as is the case in breast cancer [18].

Moreover, the exact number and definition of clinically relevant subtypes remain unclear. A recent consensus meeting agreed on the structure and features of a basal-squamous-like subtype, which is characterized by the high expression of the keratins KRT5/6 and KRT14 as well as the low expression of the transcription factors FOXA1 and GATA3 [19], which are suggested to drive luminal cell biology in bladder cancer [20]. However, to date, there has been no agreement on the definition of other non-basal subtypes or the markers necessary to define them.

Recently, using a 36-gene panel quantified by NanoString nCounter (NanoString Technologies Germany GmbH, Hamburg, Germany) in patients with MIBC treated with radical cystectomy, we were able to discriminate three prognostically distinct molecular subtypes (basal, luminal, and infiltrated) [21]. In an attempt to further reduce the required marker panel, we previously analyzed the prognostic relevance of the mRNA expression of KRT5 and KRT20 as surrogate markers for the basal and luminal subtypes of UCB, respectively [22,23]. However, it remains unclear if such a reduced marker panel adequately mirrors subtypes defined by larger marker panels.

In the present study, we investigated the association of the mRNA expression of suggested surrogate markers for the basal (KRT5) and luminal (FOXA1, GATA3, KRT20, androgen receptor (AR)) subtypes of MIBC with clinical and pathological characteristics and survival. Furthermore, the association of the surrogate markers with the subtypes defined by the previously established 36-gene panel was examined with the intent to reduce marker panels for the non-basal subtypes [21].

2. Materials and Methods

2.1. Patient Population and Histological Assessment

In this study, we retrospectively analyzed tissue samples and clinical data from 80 patients with MIBC (stage pT2–pT4) who were treated between 1998 and 2006 with radical cystectomy and bilateral lymphadenectomy at the Department of Urology of the Medical Faculty Mannheim (Mannheim, Germany). Only patients who were treated with curative intention were included. All patients with metastases (*n* = 7) or unresectable (*n* = 1) tumors at the time of diagnosis were excluded, leaving a total of 73 patients to be included in this analysis. None of the patients received neoadjuvant or adjuvant therapy. The median follow-up time was 24 months (range: 1–184 months). All patients gave written informed consent. The study was approved by the relevant institutional review board at the Medical Faculty Mannheim under numbers 2013-517N-MA and 2016-814R-MA. Hematoxylin-eosin stained sections of the tumor samples were evaluated for pathological stage according to the 2010 TNM classification and were graded according to the common grading systems (WHO 1973, WHO 2016) by an experienced uropathologist (AH).

Expression data and clinicopathological information from the publicly available cancer genome atlas network (TCGA) cohort were used for validation (*n* = 406) [14]. Only patients with MIBC (T2–T4) were included, while all patients with no documented T or N stage and patients who received neoadjuvant therapy were excluded, leaving a total of 365 patients to be included in the analysis. Based on gene expression, the samples were clustered into five molecular subtypes (basal-squamous, luminal, luminal-papillary, luminal-infiltrated, and neuronal) [24].

2.2. Assessment of mRNA Expression by RT-qPCR

A reverse transcription quantitative real-time polymerase chain reaction (RT-qPCR)-based assessment was used for the objective quantification of FOXA1, GATA3, and AR mRNA expression, as previously described and performed with KRT5 and KRT20 [22,25]. In brief, RNA was extracted from a single 10-µm section of formalin-fixed paraffin embedded (FFPE) routine tissue using a commercially available bead-based extraction method (Xtract® kit; STRATIFYER Molecular Pathology GmbH, Cologne, Germany). After a lysation and purification process, the nucleic acids were eluted and treated with DNase I. After the DNA was digested, the RNA eluates were stored at −80 °C until use.

One-step RT-qPCR was applied for the relative quantification of the mRNA expression of the genes of interest (FOXA1, GATA3 and AR) as well as the reference gene (Calmodulin 2 (CALM2)) by gene-specific TaqMan®-based assays using the SuperScript III PLATINUM One-Step, quantitative RT-PCR System (Invitrogen, Karlsruhe, Germany) on a Stratagene Mx3005p system (Agilent Technologies, Böblingen, Germany) with 30 minutes at 50 °C, two minutes at 95 °C, followed by 40 cycles of 15 seconds at 95 °C and 30 seconds at 60 °C as described previously [22,25].

Forty amplification cycles were applied, and the cycle threshold (Ct) values of the genes of interest and CALM2 for each sample were estimated as the mean value of the duplicate measurements. Ct values were then normalized against the mean expression levels of CALM2 using the 40-ΔCt method to ensure that normalized gene expression obtained by the test was proportional to the corresponding mRNA expression levels.

A set of 36 genes was previously quantified in 28 patients of this cohort using standard nCounter chemistry as previously described [21]. The nCounter assay was normalized using the geometric mean of six reference genes (CALM2, RPL37A, B2M, TUBB, GAPDH, and G6PD) and six internal positive controls, while negative background subtraction was conducted by eight negative internal controls, as previously described. Based on gene expression, urothelial carcinomas were assigned to one of three subtypes (basal, luminal, or infiltrated) [21]. Because of the small cohort size of 28 patients with available data on expression of the 36-gene panel, the subtypes were dichotomized into basal and non-basal subtypes.

The datasets for the TCGA cohort were downloaded as processed data from the open access cBioPortal database (http://www.cbioportal.org/study?id=blca_tcga#clinical) provided by the Memorial Sloan Kettering Cancer Center (New York, NY, USA). Gene expression analyses were based on paired-end RNA-Seq analysis on an Illumina HiSeq. All RSEM (RNA-Seq by Expectation Maximization) values were log2 transformed [24].

2.3. Statistical Methods

Correlation between variables was investigated by Spearman's rank correlation coefficient, Wilcoxon/Kruskal–Wallis test, or Fisher's exact test, whichever was appropriate. In addition, the cohort was stratified into patients with high or low marker expression using the median mRNA expression of KRT5, KRT20, FOXA1, GATA3, and AR as objective cut-offs. Recurrence-free survival (RFS), disease-free survival (DFS), and overall survival (OS) were analyzed by the Kaplan–Meier method and log-rank test. Univariable and multivariable analyses were performed by a Cox proportional hazards regression model. Receiver operating characteristic (ROC) curve analyses were used to measure the correlation between the markers and molecular subtypes.

Statistical analysis was performed with JMP SAS 13.0 (SAS Institute, Cary, NC, USA) or Graph Pad Prism 5 (GraphPad Software Inc., La Jolla, CA, USA). All p-values were two-sided, and a p-value <0.05 was considered to be significant.

3. Results

3.1. Association of the Surrogate Markers with Clinicopathological Features

The characteristics of the included patients are summarized in Table 1. The median mRNA expression of all analyzed markers is shown in Figure 1.

Table 1. Patient characteristics of the Mannheim cohort.

Patient Characteristic	n (%)
Tumor stage	
T2	18 (24.7)
T3	43 (58.9)
T4	12 (16.4)
Nodal status	
N0	44 (60.3)
N positive	29 (39.7)
Sex	
male	54 (74.0)
female	19 (26.0)
Grade (WHO 1973)	
G2	15 (20.5)
G3	58 (79.5)
Age	
<70	47 (64.4)
≥70	26 (35.6)
Histology	
Pure urothelial carcinoma	43 (58.9)
Histologic variants	30 (41.1)
Squamous cell	10 (13.7)
Sarcomatoid	7 (9.6)
Micropapillary	5 (6.9)
Small cell	3 (4.1)
Adenocarcinoma	2 (2.7)
Neuroendocrine	1 (1.4)
Nested	1 (1.4)
Plasmacytoid	1 (1.4)

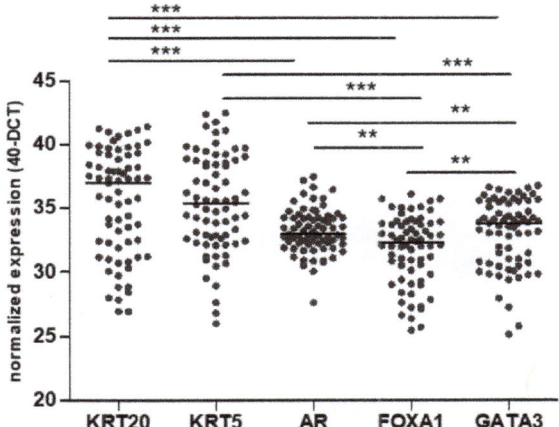

Figure 1. Distribution of normalized mRNA expression of KRT5, KRT20, FOXA1, GATA3, and androgen receptor (AR) in the Mannheim cohort (** $p < 0.01$; *** $p < 0.001$).

Spearman correlation demonstrated a significant positive association of FOXA1 and GATA3 with the luminal marker KRT20 (Figure 2). All three luminal markers showed a significantly negative association with the basal marker KRT5. Moreover, AR also showed a significantly positive association with all luminal markers, while the association between AR and KRT5 was negative.

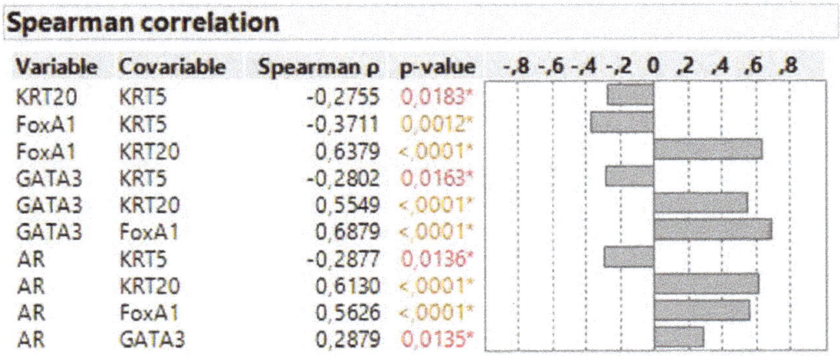

Spearman correlation				
Variable	Covariable	Spearman ρ	p-value	-.8 -.6 -.4 -.2 0 .2 .4 .6 .8
KRT20	KRT5	-0,2755	0,0183*	
FoxA1	KRT5	-0,3711	0,0012*	
FoxA1	KRT20	0,6379	<,0001*	
GATA3	KRT5	-0,2802	0,0163*	
GATA3	KRT20	0,5549	<,0001*	
GATA3	FoxA1	0,6879	<,0001*	
AR	KRT5	-0,2877	0,0136*	
AR	KRT20	0,6130	<,0001*	
AR	FoxA1	0,5626	<,0001*	
AR	GATA3	0,2879	0,0135*	

Figure 2. Spearman correlation of all measured markers (* $p < 0.05$).

The Wilcoxon/Kruskal–Wallis test showed significant positive associations between grade and both KRT5 (0.0388) and GATA3 ($p = 0.0133$). There were no significant associations with tumor stage, nodal status, sex, or age.

3.2. Association of the Surrogate Markers with Survival

For survival analysis, the median mRNA expression levels of each marker were used as an objective cut-off to stratify patients with high and low marker expression. Kaplan–Meier analysis indicated that high KRT20 ($p = 0.0317$) and FOXA1 ($p = 0.0048$) expression was associated with significantly reduced RFS. GATA3 ($p = 0.0629$) and KRT5 ($p = 0.0513$) were not significantly associated with RFS. When analyzing the association with DFS and OS, only FOXA1 was significantly associated with reduced DFS ($p = 0.0186$) (Figure 3), while KRT5, KRT20, and GATA3 showed no associations with OS or DFS. AR mRNA expression showed no relevant associations with RFS, DFS, or OS.

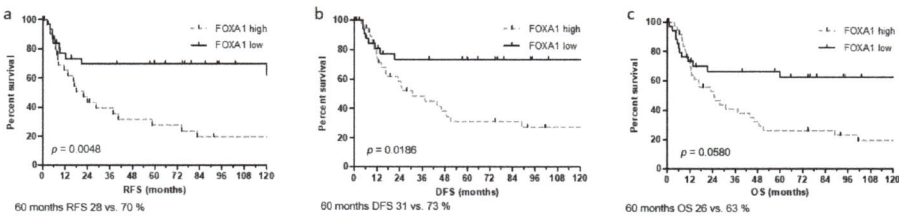

Figure 3. Kaplan Meier analysis for recurrence-free survival (RFS) (**a**), disease-free survival (DFS) (**b**) and overall survival (OS) (**c**) based on FOXA1 mRNA expression within the Mannheim cohort.

In univariable Cox regression analysis, positive nodal status, tumor stage, and expression of FOXA1 and KRT20 were associated with worse outcome (Tables 2–4). In the multivariable analysis, of all examined markers, only FOXA1 remained an independent prognostic marker for DFS ($p = 0.0333$) and RFS ($p = 0.0310$) (Tables 2–4). When analyzing patients with pure urothelial carcinomas ($n = 43$) and patients with histologic variants ($n = 30$) separately, we found an improved survival for patients with low FOXA1 expression and pure urothelial carcinomas but not histologic variants, which might be attributed to the low number of 30 patients and high heterogeneity of the histologic variants (Figure S1).

Table 2. Univariable and multivariable Cox regression analyses for RFS (Recurrence-free survival), accounting for all five analyzed markers and clinicopathological features.

Parameter	Univariable		Multivariable	
	Hazard Ratio	*p*-Value	Hazard Ratio	*p*-Value
Tumor stage T3/4 vs. T2	1.6203	0.2156		
Nodal status N+ vs. N0	2.8737	**0.0027**	2.4330	**0.0146**
Sex male vs. female	1.0155	0.9698		
Grade (WHO 1973) G2 vs. G3	0.4709	0.8186		
Age <70 vs. ≥70	0.8428	0.6454		
KRT5 >median vs. <median	0.5081	0.0513		
KRT20 >median vs. <median	2.1233	**0.0317**	1.2927	0.5083
FOXA1 >median vs. <median	2.7209	**0.0048**	2.2670	**0.0310**
GATA3 >median vs. <median	1.9211	0.0629		
AR >median vs. <median	1.6121	0.1670		

Multivariable analysis was performed only for significant parameters in univariable analysis (significant values in bold).

Table 3. Univariable and multivariable Cox regression analyses for DFS (Disease-free survival), accounting for all five analyzed markers and clinicopathological features.

Parameter	Univariable		Multivariable	
	Hazard Ratio	p-Value	Hazard Ratio	p-Value
Tumor stage T3/4 vs. T2	2.0330	0.0926		
Nodal status N+ vs. N0	2.7727	**0.0044**	2.6057	**0.0077**
Sex male vs. female	1.5435	0.2715		
Grade (WHO 1973) G2 G3	1.1484	0.7558		
Age <70 ≥70	0.8833	0.7404		
KRT5 >median vs. <median	0.6999	0.3072		
KRT20 >median vs. <median	1.3249	0.4235		
FOXA1 >median vs. <median	2.3617	**0.0186**	2.1946	**0.0333**
GATA3 >median vs. <median	1.2429	0.5359		
AR >median vs. <median	1.3717	0.3670		

Multivariable analysis was performed only for significant parameters in univariable analysis (significant values in bold).

There was no association between FOXA1 expression and DFS in the TCGA cohort (Figure S2).

3.3. Correlation of Surrogate Markers with Molecular Subtypes Defined by Multigene Panels

In the Mannheim cohort, a total of 28 patients were clustered into three molecular subtypes (basal, luminal, and infiltrated) according to the expression of a 36-gene panel previously quantified with nCounter [21]. Because of the small cohort with available data on molecular subtypes, we dichotomized the subtypes into basal and non-basal subtypes in the present study. The Mann–Whitney test showed that FOXA1 ($p = 0.0028$) and KRT20 ($p = 0.011$) expression was significantly higher in the non-basal subtype (Figure 4). The expression of KRT5 ($p = 0.083$) and GATA3 ($p = 0.11$) was not significantly different between the two subtypes in the Mannheim cohort. In the TCGA cohort, all three luminal markers had significantly higher expression in the non-basal subtype, while KRT5 was significantly higher in the basal subtype (each $p < 0.0001$).

Table 4. Univariable and multivariable Cox regression analyses for OS (Overall survival), accounting for all five analyzed markers and clinicopathological features.

Parameter	Univariable		Multivariable	
	Hazard Ratio	p-Value	Hazard Ratio	p-Value
Tumor stage T3/4 vs. T2	2.0601	**0.0048**	1.7819	0.1251
Nodal status N+ vs. N0	2.2720	**0.0086**	2.0806	**0.0206**
Sex male vs. female	1.3586	0.3820		
Grade (WHO 1973) G2 vs. G3	0.7678	0.4590		
Age <70 vs. ≥70	0.8253	0.5544		
KRT5 >median vs. <median	0.7012	0.2408		
KRT20 >median vs. <median	1.1560	0.6334		
FOXA1 >median vs. <median	1.7986	0.0580		
GATA3 >median vs. <median	1.0844	0.7800		
AR >median vs. <median	1.3104	0.3728		

Multivariable analysis was performed only for significant parameters in univariable analysis (significant values in bold).

Using the median marker expression as the cut-off, ROC analyses showed a high but not significant correlation of KRT5 with the basal subtype (AUC = 0.65; p = 0.097) in the Mannheim cohort. FOXA1 (AUC = 0.79; p = 0.0007) and KRT20 (AUC = 0.75; p = 0.0066) correlated significantly with the non-basal subtype, unlike GATA3 (AUC = 0.65; p = 0.097). The use of all three luminal markers combined showed no relevantly improved approximation to the non-basal subtype (AUC = 0.79; p = 0.0015) over the use of KRT20 or especially FOXA1 alone. Validation in the TCGA cohort showed that the use of FOXA1 alone (AUC = 0.77; p < 0.0001) achieved a high approximation to the non-basal subtype, similar to the use of all three markers combined (AUC = 0.79; p < 0.0001), while KRT5 achieved a close approximation to the basal subtype (AUC = 0.75; p < 0.0001). To exclude the possibility that the high association of KRT5 and FOXA1 with the basal and non-basal subtypes is mainly based on the central role of KRT5 and FOXA1 in the classification of subtypes using the 36-gene panel and the TCGA classification, we applied the BASE47 signature, which does not include KRT5 and FOXA1 for defining subtypes, on the TCGA cohort for validation [16]. This way, KRT5 and FOXA1 still showed a significantly higher distribution in the basal and luminal subtype, respectively (Figure S3). Furthermore, there was still a high association between the basal subtype and KRT5 (AUC = 0.72; $p < 0.0001$) and the luminal subtype and FOXA1 (AUC = 0.77; $p < 0.0001$).

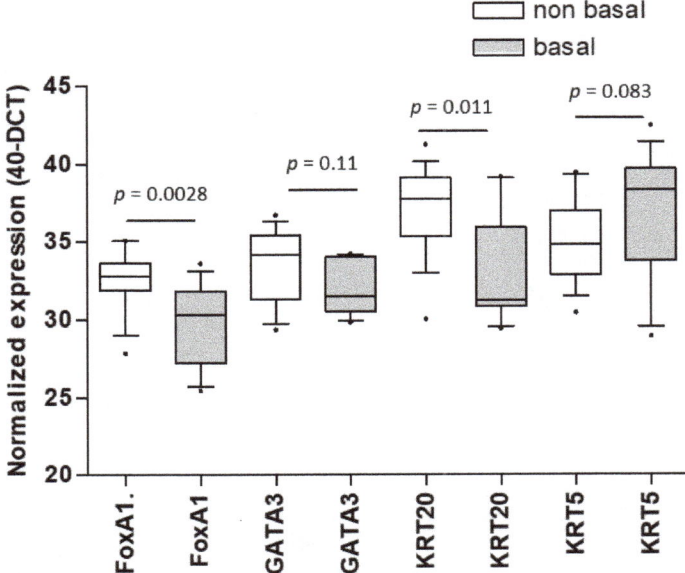

Figure 4. Distribution of FOXA1, GATA3, KRT20, and KRT5 within the basal and non-basal subtypes defined by a 36-gene panel within the Mannheim cohort showing significantly higher expression of FOXA1 and KRT20 in the non-basal subtype.

4. Discussion

With the advent of molecular subtyping in UCB, researchers and clinicians are faced with several problems, as was the case with molecular subtyping in breast cancer 15 years ago. First, apart from a basal squamous-like subtype, no consensus on the number and essential characteristics of other molecular subtypes has yet been reached [19]. As most groups have defined various numbers of luminal-like subtypes, these differences in labeling, subclassification and marker expression have hindered the general acceptance of these non-basal subtypes so far [12,14,16,21].

Second, it is necessary that subtypes are either prognostically or therapeutically relevant; otherwise, they are useless for daily clinical routine. For instance, analogous to breast cancer, a claudin-low subset of basal UCB was previously defined which demonstrated a similar outcome as regular basal UCB [16], therefore being of no interest for clinical routine.

Third, the analysis of hundreds of genes per patient currently used by most groups for the definition of their subtypes is too time-consuming and cost-intensive for easy transfer into a routine clinical setting, which is why a small set of surrogate markers per subtype has to be determined. In breast cancer, it was shown that the analysis of only four markers (estrogen receptor, progesterone receptor, HER2, and Ki-67) is enough to make a valid therapeutically relevant molecular classification [18,26]. In addition, a recent study in prostate cancer showed that the status of the PTEN gene alone matched a multigene panel to predict the risk of metastasis in patients treated with radical prostatectomy, allowing for more cost-saving diagnostics [27].

By analogy to previous findings in breast and prostate cancer, the goal of the present study was to identify surrogate markers for molecular subtypes with regard to their prognostic relevance and concordance with subtypes defined by multigene panels. Given that there is consensus about the basal subtype, we focused on non-basal subtypes. Therefore, we decided to analyze the mRNA expression of the two prominent luminal markers, FOXA1 and GATA3, together with the previously measured luminal marker KRT20 and the basal marker KRT5 [22], alongside AR as a potential target associated with the luminal subtype of MIBC [28].

Regarding the expression pattern, our results are in concordance with previous findings, as FOXA1 and GATA3 are strongly associated with KRT20 expression and show a negative association with KRT5 [12,16]. As before, we found AR to be associated with the luminal subtype in MIBC [28].

When comparing single-marker analysis to the subtypes defined by the 36-gene panel, FOXA1 and KRT20 expression was significantly higher in the non-basal subtype than in the basal subtype. Moreover, the analysis of only FOXA1 or KRT20 showed a similar high correlation with the 36-gene panel when compared to the analysis of FOXA1, GATA3 and KRT20 combined. The use of FOXA1 alone showed an almost identical AUC in the Mannheim (0.79) and TCGA (0.77) cohorts when compared to the use of all three luminal markers together (Mannheim 0.79; TCGA 0.76). FOXA1 is known to play a central role in urothelial differentiation. In addition, the low expression or loss of FOXA1 in basal tumors was described in the development of squamous cell carcinoma in preclinical models of bladder cancer, which is in concordance with the subtype association in the current study [29]. The nonsignificant correlation of GATA3 with the non-basal subtype and KRT5 with the basal subtype in the Mannheim cohort might be attributed to the small sample size of only 28 patients for whom the 36-gene panel results were available. The correlation of all markers with their respective subtype was confirmed in the TCGA cohort. The current results indicate that the measurement of one of the luminal markers, could be enough to determine a non-basal subtype, potentially allowing for more cost-saving diagnostics in daily clinical routine.

When analyzing the prognostic relevance, high KRT5 showed a non-significant trend for prolonged RFS, while FOXA1 was the only luminal marker that remained an independent prognostic marker for reduced RFS when all markers were accounted for, which suggests that a combined analysis of all three luminal markers does not provide any additional prognostically relevant information. These results are in contrast to several previous studies that found the basal subtype to be associated with worse outcome [15,17]. With regard to FOXA1 in particular, Yuk and colleagues reported higher FOXA1 expression to be associated with a positive prognostic outcome using immunohistochemistry on tissue microarray slides [30]. One possible reason for this discrepancy might be the high percentage (41%) of histologic variants within the analyzed Mannheim cohort, which are often associated with poorer prognosis than pure urothelial carcinomas and demonstrate a higher expression of luminal markers such as FOXA1 [20,31]. Furthermore, some studies show an association between the high expression of luminal markers such as KRT20 and high tumor stage, grade and micrometastasis, which are known to be associated with worse survival, which further indicates a luminal patient group with impaired survival [32,33]. On the other hand, no prognostic relevance for any of the luminal markers could be shown in the TCGA cohort. Tumor heterogeneity, which was not accounted for in the current study, might also be a factor for these contradictory results [34]. Further studies are necessary to clarify the prognostic role of molecular markers in MIBC.

Moreover, while the analysis of only one basal and one luminal marker seems to be enough to make a valid distinction between the basal and non-basal subtypes, additional markers still might be necessary for subclassification. In a comprehensive molecular analysis of MIBC within the TCGA cohort, Robertson et al. were able to identify three distinct luminal subclasses, with the luminal and luminal-infiltrated subtypes being associated with reduced survival compared to the luminal-papillary subtype [24]. All three luminal subtypes showed comparable expression patterns of FOXA1, GATA3, and KRT20 but differed with regard to FGFR3 mutations, lymphocytic infiltration, smooth muscle gene signatures, and uroplakin expression. Differences in luminal subclasses were not accounted for in our current study. The analysis of one or two additional markers (for instance, the epithelial–mesenchymal transition (EMT) markers TWIST1 or SNAI1) might be enough to draw clinically relevant conclusions. Moreover, a rare neuronal/neuroendocrine-like subtype associated with poor survival has previously been described in approximately 5% of patients with MIBC [24,35]. These tumors are mainly characterized by the upregulation of genes of neuroendocrine origin, such as TUBB2B but can also express FOXA1 and GATA3. Markers to distinguish these neuronal/neuroendocrine-like subtypes from luminal subtypes still have to be defined.

As previously mentioned, with a total of 73 included patients, our cohort is relatively small compared to other multicentric studies. On the other hand, given that this is a single center study, we have exact information on treatment modalities, which is necessary to interpret the prognostic relevance of markers, although some data on salvage therapies is missing due to the retrospective nature of the study. However, this is also the case in the TCGA cohort, where no precise information on the treatment modality is provided, rendering statements about prognosis even more difficult.

5. Conclusions

In conclusion, we were able to demonstrate that the measurement of only one of the prominent luminal markers alongside KRT5 as the basal marker is enough to make a valid distinction between the basal and non-basal subtypes and potentially draw prognostically relevant conclusions. Given the closest concordance with subtypes defined by multigene panels as well as strongest prognostic relevance, FOXA1 seems to be the marker best suited as a surrogate marker to distinguish the non-basal subtypes from the basal subtypes. The measurement of FOXA1, GATA3, and KRT20 combined does not provide any additional relevant information. However, additional studies are necessary to further clarify the prognostic role of molecular markers in MIBC. Moreover, surrogate markers for the further subclassification of the luminal subtype still have to be defined.

Supplementary Materials: The following are available online at http://www.mdpi.com/2077-0383/9/4/994/s1, Figure S1: Kaplan–Meier analysis for RFS, DFS, and OS based on FOXA1 mRNA expression within the Mannheim cohort in patients with pure urothelial carcinoma and patients with histologic variants. Figure S2: Kaplan–Meier analysis for disease specific survival based on FOXA1 mRNA expression within the TCGA cohort. Figure S3: Distribution of normalized mRNA expression of FOXA1 within the basal and luminal subtypes defined by a 47-gene panel (BASE47) within the TCGA cohort.

Author Contributions: Conceptualization: D.S., R.M.W., B.K., C.B., B.W., and P.E.; Methodology, D.S., M.E, R.M.W., J.J., S.P., V.W., S.R., A.H., and P.E.; Validation: M.E., T.S.W., F.K., V.W., J.B., W.O., S.R., C.B., and B.W.; Formal Analysis: D.S., R.M.W., A.H., and P.E.; Investigation, D.S., R.M.W., J.B., and P.E.; Data Curation: D.S., J.J., T.S.W., S.P., and P.E.; Writing—Original Draft Preparation: D.S., B.K., J.B., B.W., and P.E.; Writing—Review and Editing: D.S., M.E., J.J., T.S.W., F.K., V.W., J.B., W.O., S.R., C.B., A.H., and P.E.; Visualization: D.S., R.M.W., and P.E.; Supervision: T.S.W., S.P., B.K., F.K., W.O., S.R., C.B., A.H., and B.W.; Project Administration: D.S. and P.E. All authors have read and agreed to the published version of the manuscript.

Funding: This research received no external funding.

Acknowledgments: D.S. is supported by a Ferdinand Eisenberger grant from the German Society of Urology (Deutsche Gesellschaft für Urologie), grant ID SiD1/FE-16.

Conflicts of Interest: R.M.W. is a founder of STRATIFYER Molecular Pathology GmbH. The other authors declare no conflicts of interest.

References

1. Bray, F.; Ferlay, J.; Soerjomataram, I.; Siegel, R.L.; Torre, L.A.; Jemal, A. Global cancer statistics 2018: GLOBOCAN estimates of incidence and mortality worldwide for 36 cancers in 185 countries. *CA A Cancer J. Clin.* **2018**, *68*, 394–424. [CrossRef] [PubMed]
2. Burger, M.; Catto, J.W.; Dalbagni, G.; Grossman, H.B.; Herr, H.; Karakiewicz, P.; Kassouf, W.; Kiemeney, L.A.; La Vecchia, C.; Shariat, S.; et al. Epidemiology and risk factors of urothelial bladder cancer. *Eur. Urol.* **2013**, *63*, 234–241. [CrossRef] [PubMed]
3. Alfred Witjes, J.; Lebret, T.; Comperat, E.M.; Cowan, N.C.; De Santis, M.; Bruins, H.M.; Hernandez, V.; Espinos, E.L.; Dunn, J.; Rouanne, M.; et al. Updated 2016 EAU Guidelines on Muscle-invasive and Metastatic Bladder Cancer. *Eur. Urol.* **2017**, *71*, 462–475. [CrossRef] [PubMed]
4. Babjuk, M.; Bohle, A.; Burger, M.; Capoun, O.; Cohen, D.; Comperat, E.M.; Hernandez, V.; Kaasinen, E.; Palou, J.; Roupret, M.; et al. EAU Guidelines on Non-Muscle-invasive Urothelial Carcinoma of the Bladder: Update 2016. *Eur. Urol.* **2017**, *71*, 447–461. [CrossRef] [PubMed]

5. Aziz, A.; Gierth, M.; Rink, M.; Schmid, M.; Chun, F.K.; Dahlem, R.; Roghmann, F.; Palisaar, R.J.; Noldus, J.; Ellinger, J.; et al. Optimizing outcome reporting after radical cystectomy for organ-confined urothelial carcinoma of the bladder using oncological trifecta and pentafecta. *World J. Urol.* **2015**, *33*, 1945–1950. [CrossRef] [PubMed]
6. Donat, S.M. Staged based directed surveillance of invasive bladder cancer following radical cystectomy: Valuable and effective? *World J. Urol.* **2006**, *24*, 557–564. [CrossRef] [PubMed]
7. Hassan, J.M.; Cookson, M.S.; Smith, J.A., Jr.; Chang, S.S. Patterns of initial transitional cell recurrence in patients after cystectomy. *J. Urol.* **2006**, *175*, 2054–2057. [CrossRef]
8. Yoo, S.H.; Kim, H.; Kwak, C.; Kim, H.H.; Jung, J.H.; Ku, J.H. Late Recurrence of Bladder Cancer following Radical Cystectomy: Characteristics and Outcomes. *Urol. Int.* **2019**, *103*, 1–6. [CrossRef]
9. Svatek, R.S.; Hollenbeck, B.K.; Holmang, S.; Lee, R.; Kim, S.P.; Stenzl, A.; Lotan, Y. The economics of bladder cancer: Costs and considerations of caring for this disease. *Eur. Urol.* **2014**, *66*, 253–262. [CrossRef]
10. Botteman, M.F.; Pashos, C.L.; Redaelli, A.; Laskin, B.; Hauser, R. The health economics of bladder cancer: A comprehensive review of the published literature. *PharmacoEconomics* **2003**, *21*, 1315–1330. [CrossRef]
11. Gore, J.L.; Gilbert, S.M. Improving bladder cancer patient care: A pharmacoeconomic perspective. *Expert Rev. Anticancer. Ther.* **2013**, *13*, 661–668. [CrossRef]
12. Choi, W.; Porten, S.; Kim, S.; Willis, D.; Plimack, E.R.; Hoffman-Censits, J.; Roth, B.; Cheng, T.; Tran, M.; Lee, I.-L.; et al. Identification of distinct basal and luminal subtypes of muscle-invasive bladder cancer with different sensitivities to frontline chemotherapy. *Cancer Cell* **2014**, *25*, 152–165. [CrossRef] [PubMed]
13. Sjödahl, G.; Lauss, M.; Lövgren, K.; Chebil, G.; Gudjonsson, S.; Veerla, S.; Patschan, O.; Aine, M.; Fernö, M.; Ringnér, M.; et al. A molecular taxonomy for urothelial carcinoma. *Clin. Cancer Res.* **2012**, *18*, 3377–3386. [CrossRef] [PubMed]
14. Network, C.G.A.R. Comprehensive molecular characterization of urothelial bladder carcinoma. *Nature* **2014**, *507*, 315–322. [CrossRef]
15. Choi, W.; Czerniak, B.; Ochoa, A.; Su, X.; Siefker-Radtke, A.; Dinney, C.; McConkey, D.J. Intrinsic basal and luminal subtypes of muscle-invasive bladder cancer. *Nat. Rev. Urol.* **2014**, *11*, 400–410. [CrossRef]
16. Damrauer, J.S.; Hoadley, K.A.; Chism, D.D.; Fan, C.; Tiganelli, C.J.; Wobker, S.E.; Yeh, J.J.; Milowsky, M.I.; Iyer, G.; Parker, J.S.; et al. Intrinsic subtypes of high-grade bladder cancer reflect the hallmarks of breast cancer biology. *Proc. Natl. Acad. Sci. USA* **2014**, *111*, 3110–3115. [CrossRef]
17. Seiler, R.; Ashab, H.A.D.; Erho, N.; van Rhijn, B.W.G.; Winters, B.; Douglas, J.; Van Kessel, K.E.; Fransen van de Putte, E.E.; Sommerlad, M.; Wang, N.Q.; et al. Impact of Molecular Subtypes in Muscle-invasive Bladder Cancer on Predicting Response and Survival after Neoadjuvant Chemotherapy. *Eur. Urol.* **2017**, *72*, 544–554. [CrossRef]
18. Goldhirsch, A.; Wood, W.C.; Coates, A.S.; Gelber, R.D.; Thurlimann, B.; Senn, H.J.; Panel, M. Strategies for subtypes–dealing with the diversity of breast cancer: Highlights of the St. Gallen International Expert Consensus on the Primary Therapy of Early Breast Cancer 2011. *Ann. Oncol.* **2011**, *22*, 1736–1747. [CrossRef]
19. Lerner, S.P.; McConkey, D.J.; Hoadley, K.A.; Chan, K.S.; Kim, W.Y.; Radvanyi, F.; Hoglund, M.; Real, F.X. Bladder Cancer Molecular Taxonomy: Summary from a Consensus Meeting. *Bladder Cancer* **2016**, *2*, 37–47. [CrossRef]
20. Warrick, J.I.; Kaag, M.; Raman, J.D.; Chan, W.; Tran, T.; Kunchala, S.; Shuman, L.; DeGraff, D.; Chen, G. FOXA1 and CK14 as markers of luminal and basal subtypes in histologic variants of bladder cancer and their associated conventional urothelial carcinoma. *Virchows Arch. Int. J. Pathol.* **2017**, *471*, 337–345. [CrossRef]
21. Rinaldetti, S.; Rempel, E.; Worst, T.S.; Eckstein, M.; Steidler, A.; Weiss, C.A.; Bolenz, C.; Hartmann, A.; Erben, P. Subclassification, survival prediction and drug target analyses of chemotherapy-naive muscle-invasive bladder cancer with a molecular screening. *Oncotarget* **2018**, *9*, 25935–25945. [CrossRef] [PubMed]
22. Eckstein, M.; Wirtz, R.M.; Gross-Weege, M.; Breyer, J.; Otto, W.; Stoehr, R.; Sikic, D.; Keck, B.; Eidt, S.; Burger, M.; et al. mRNA-Expression of KRT5 and KRT20 Defines Distinct Prognostic Subgroups of Muscle-Invasive Urothelial Bladder Cancer Correlating with Histological Variants. *Int. J. Mol. Sci.* **2018**, *19*, 3396. [CrossRef] [PubMed]
23. Breyer, J.; Wirtz, R.M.; Otto, W.; Erben, P.; Kriegmair, M.C.; Stoehr, R.; Eckstein, M.; Eidt, S.; Denzinger, S.; Burger, M.; et al. In stage pT1 non-muscle-invasive bladder cancer (NMIBC), high KRT20 and low KRT5 mRNA expression identify the luminal subtype and predict recurrence and survival. *Virchows Arch. Int. J. Pathol.* **2017**, *470*, 267–274. [CrossRef]

24. Robertson, A.G.; Kim, J.; Al-Ahmadie, H.; Bellmunt, J.; Guo, G.; Cherniack, A.D.; Hinoue, T.; Laird, P.W.; Hoadley, K.A.; Akbani, R.; et al. Comprehensive Molecular Characterization of Muscle-Invasive Bladder Cancer. *Cell* **2017**, *171*, 540–556.e55. [CrossRef] [PubMed]
25. Breyer, J.; Otto, W.; Wirtz, R.M.; Wullich, B.; Keck, B.; Erben, P.; Kriegmair, M.C.; Stoehr, R.; Eckstein, M.; Laible, M.; et al. ERBB2 Expression as Potential Risk-Stratification for Early Cystectomy in Patients with pT1 Bladder Cancer and Concomitant Carcinoma in situ. *Urol. Int.* **2016**. [CrossRef] [PubMed]
26. Perou, C.M.; Sorlie, T.; Eisen, M.B.; van de Rijn, M.; Jeffrey, S.S.; Rees, C.A.; Pollack, J.R.; Ross, D.T.; Johnsen, H.; Akslen, L.A.; et al. Molecular portraits of human breast tumours. *Nature* **2000**, *406*, 747–752. [CrossRef] [PubMed]
27. Leapman, M.S.; Nguyen, H.G.; Cowan, J.E.; Xue, L.; Stohr, B.; Simko, J.; Cooperberg, M.R.; Carroll, P.R. Comparing Prognostic Utility of a Single-marker Immunohistochemistry Approach with Commercial Gene Expression Profiling Following Radical Prostatectomy. *Eur. Urol.* **2018**, *74*, 668–675. [CrossRef]
28. Sikic, D.; Wirtz, R.M.; Wach, S.; Dyrskjot, L.; Erben, P.; Bolenz, C.; Breyer, J.; Otto, W.; Hoadley, K.A.; Lerner, S.P.; et al. Androgen Receptor mRNA Expression in Urothelial Carcinoma of the Bladder: A Retrospective Analysis of Two Independent Cohorts. *Transl. Oncol.* **2019**, *12*, 661–668. [CrossRef]
29. DeGraff, D.J.; Clark, P.E.; Cates, J.M.; Yamashita, H.; Robinson, V.L.; Yu, X.; Smolkin, M.E.; Chang, S.S.; Cookson, M.S.; Herrick, M.K.; et al. Loss of the urothelial differentiation marker FOXA1 is associated with high grade, late stage bladder cancer and increased tumor proliferation. *PLoS ONE* **2012**, *7*, e36669. [CrossRef]
30. Yuk, H.D.; Jeong, C.W.; Kwak, C.; Kim, H.H.; Moon, K.C.; Ku, J.H. Clinical outcomes of muscle invasive bladder Cancer according to the BASQ classification. *BMC Cancer* **2019**, *19*, 897. [CrossRef]
31. Lopez-Beltran, A.; Henriques, V.; Montironi, R. Variants and new entities of bladder cancer. *Histopathology* **2019**, *74*, 77–96. [CrossRef] [PubMed]
32. Christoph, F.; Muller, M.; Schostak, M.; Soong, R.; Tabiti, K.; Miller, K. Quantitative detection of cytokeratin 20 mRNA expression in bladder carcinoma by real-time reverse transcriptase-polymerase chain reaction. *Urology* **2004**, *64*, 157–161. [CrossRef] [PubMed]
33. Gazquez, C.; Ribal, M.J.; Marin-Aguilera, M.; Kayed, H.; Fernandez, P.L.; Mengual, L.; Alcaraz, A. Biomarkers vs conventional histological analysis to detect lymph node micrometastases in bladder cancer: A real improvement? *BJU Int.* **2012**, *110*, 1310–1316. [CrossRef] [PubMed]
34. Thomsen, M.B.H.; Nordentoft, I.; Lamy, P.; Vang, S.; Reinert, L.; Mapendano, C.K.; Hoyer, S. Comprehensive multiregional analysis of molecular heterogeneity in bladder cancer. *Sci. Rep.* **2017**, *7*, 11702. [CrossRef] [PubMed]
35. Sjodahl, G.; Eriksson, P.; Liedberg, F.; Hoglund, M. Molecular classification of urothelial carcinoma: Global mRNA classification versus tumour-cell phenotype classification. *J. Pathol.* **2017**, *242*, 113–125. [CrossRef]

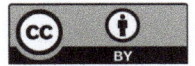

© 2020 by the authors. Licensee MDPI, Basel, Switzerland. This article is an open access article distributed under the terms and conditions of the Creative Commons Attribution (CC BY) license (http://creativecommons.org/licenses/by/4.0/).

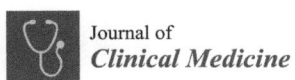

Article

A Multiplex Test Assessing $MiR663a_{me}$ and VIM_{me} in Urine Accurately Discriminates Bladder Cancer from Inflammatory Conditions

Sara Monteiro-Reis [1], Ana Blanca [2], Joana Tedim-Moreira [1], Isa Carneiro [1,3], Diana Montezuma [1,3], Paula Monteiro [1,3], Jorge Oliveira [4], Luís Antunes [5], Rui Henrique [1,2,6], António Lopez-Beltran [7,8] and Carmen Jerónimo [1,6,*]

[1] Cancer Biology and Epigenetics Group—Research Center (CI-IPOP), Portuguese Oncology Institute of Porto (IPO Porto), and Porto Comprehensive Cancer Center (P.CCC), Maimonides Biomedical Research Institute of Cordoba, 14004 Cordoba, Spain; sara.raquel.reis@ipoporto.min-saude.pt (S.M.-R.); joana.matos@ua.pt (J.T.-M.); isa.carneiro@ipoporto.min-saude.pt (I.C.); dianafelizardo@gmail.com (D.M.); paula.monteiro@ipoporto.min-saude.pt (P.M.); henrique@ipoporto.min-saude.pt (R.H.)
[2] Department of Urology, University Hospital of Reina Sofia, Maimonides Biomedical Research Institute of Cordoba, 14004 Cordoba, Spain; anblape78@hotmail.com
[3] Department of Pathology, Portuguese Oncology Institute of Porto (IPO Porto), 4200-072 Porto, Portugal
[4] Department of Urology, Portuguese Oncology Institute of Porto (IPO-Porto), 4200-072 Porto, Portugal; jorge.oliveira@ipoporto.min-saude.pt
[5] Department of Epidemiology, Portuguese Oncology Institute of Porto (IPO Porto) & Cancer Epidemiology Group—Research Center (CI-IPOP), 4200-072 Porto, Portugal; luis.antunes@ipoporto.min-saude.pt
[6] Department of Pathology and Molecular Immunology, Institute of Biomedical Sciences Abel Salazar (ICBAS)—University of Porto, 4050-313 Porto, Portugal
[7] Department of Surgery and Pathology, Faculty of Medicine, University of Cordoba, 14071 Cordoba, Spain; em1lobea@uco.es
[8] Champalimaud Clinical Center, 1400-038 Lisbon, Portugal
* Correspondence: carmenjeronimo@ipoporto.min-saude.pt; Tel.: +35-122-508-4000

Received: 28 January 2020; Accepted: 18 February 2020; Published: 24 February 2020

Abstract: Bladder cancer (BlCa) is a common malignancy with significant morbidity and mortality. Current diagnostic methods are invasive and costly, showing the need for newer biomarkers. Although several epigenetic-based biomarkers have been proposed, their ability to discriminate BlCa from common benign conditions of the urinary tract, especially inflammatory diseases, has not been adequately explored. Herein, we sought to determine whether VIM_{me} and $miR663a_{me}$ might accurately discriminate those two conditions, using a multiplex test. Performance of VIM_{me} and $miR663a_{me}$ in tissue samples and urines in testing set confirmed previous results (96.3% sensitivity, 88.2% specificity, area under de curve (AUC) 0.98 and 92.6% sensitivity, 75% specificity, AUC 0.83, respectively). In the validation sets, VIM_{me}-$miR663a_{me}$ multiplex test in urine discriminated BlCa patients from healthy donors or patients with inflammatory conditions, with 87% sensitivity, 86% specificity and 80% sensitivity, 75% specificity, respectively. Furthermore, positive likelihood ratio (LR) of 2.41 and negative LR of 0.21 were also disclosed. Compared to urinary cytology, VIM_{me}-$miR663a_{me}$ multiplex panel correctly detected 87% of the analysed cases, whereas cytology only forecasted 41%. Furthermore, high $miR663a_{me}$ independently predicted worse clinical outcome, especially in patients with invasive BlCa. We concluded that the implementation of this panel might better stratify patients for confirmatory, invasive examinations, ultimately improving the cost-effectiveness of BlCa diagnosis and management. Moreover, $miR663a_{me}$ analysis might provide relevant information for patient monitoring, identifying patients at higher risk for cancer progression.

Keywords: bladder cancer; methylation; biomarkers

1. Introduction

Bladder cancer (BlCa) is one of the most incident cancers, ranking ninth in prevalence worldwide [1,2]. In men, which are more prone to develop BlCa, it represents the second most frequent urological malignancy after prostate cancer [1,2]. Moreover, it is expected that, by 2040, the number of estimated new cases and cancer-related deaths will almost double the 549,393 newly diagnosed cases and 199,922 deaths recorded in 2018 [1,2]. Most BlCa cases correspond to urothelial carcinoma, generally presenting as non-muscle invasive BlCa (NMIBC), accounting for 75–80% of all new cases, characterised by frequent recurrences and eventual progression to more aggressive, deeply invasive and metastatic disease, or muscle-invasive BlCa (MIBC), an aggressive, locally invading carcinoma, corresponding to 20–25% of all cases, with propensity for metastasation [3,4]. Haematuria is the most common clinical sign of BlCa, although it also occurs in several common benign disease such as urinary tract infections and non-infectious inflammatory conditions. Presently, BlCa diagnosis generally involves cytoscopic examination, an expensive and invasive procedure, complemented by urine cytology [5–7]. However, the latter has limited accuracy, particularly for identification of low-grade papillary tumours, and the invasive nature of cystoscopic examination entails patient discomfort and, in some cases, infection [5]. Moreover, because of the high incidence, recurrence and progression rate, active long follow-up is required, making BlCa the costliest malignancy [8]. Thus, early, accurate and non-invasive BlCa detection is the determinant to improve both patients and healthcare financial management.

Epigenetic changes, including DNA methylation, have been largely investigated for cancer detection [9]. Owing to chemical and biological stability, DNA methylation-based biomarkers have potential clinical applications in early cancer detection, diagnosis, follow-up and targeted therapies [10]. Previously, two independent DNA methylation-based biomarker panels have been reported as promising tests for accurate early detection of BlCa [11,12]. In 2010, a three-gene panel comprised *GDF15*, *TMEFF2* and *VIM* methylation identified BlCa with 94% sensitivity and 100% specificity in urine samples from 51 BlCa patients [11]. More recently, a panel testing the promoter methylation of two microRNAs—*miR129-2* and *miR663a*—identified urothelial carcinoma (from upper and lower urinary tracts) with a sensitivity of 87.8% and specificity of 82.7% in 49 urine samples from patients with urothelial carcinoma [12]. Furthermore, the same panels could discriminate BlCa from other common genitourinary cancers (i.e., from kidney and prostate). Nonetheless, both studies used a singleplex approach, and the ability of these tests to discriminate BlCa from common benign conditions of the urinary tract with overlapping manifestations, especially inflammatory diseases, has not been adequately explored, thus far. Indeed, inflammatory conditions of the urinary tract may negatively impact the specificity of urinary-based biomarkers for BlCa detection, increasing false positive results and entailing unnecessary complementary invasive tests [6,13,14].

Thus, we sought to assess whether the most promising markers in each published panel—*miR-663a* (*miR663a*$_{me}$) and *Vimentin* (*VIM*$_{me}$)—might accurately discriminate BlCa from inflammatory conditions in voided urine, allowing for the development of a multiplex test that could be used for early detection in clinical practice.

2. Experimental Section

2.1. Patients and Tumour Sample Collection

Ninety-four primary BlCa tissue samples were obtained from a consecutive series of patients diagnosed, treated with transurethral resection (TUR) or radical cystectomy, between 1994 and 2011, and followed at Portuguese Oncology Institute of Porto (IPO Porto), Portugal (Table 1). Briefly, tumour samples were obtained during surgery and immediately snap-frozen, stored at −80 °C and subsequently macrodissected for tumours' cells enrichment and cut in cryostat for DNA extraction. Routine collection and processing of tissue samples allowed for pathological examination, classification, grading and staging [15]. For control purposes, an independent set of 19 normal bladder mucosae

(NB) samples were also collected from BlCa-free individuals (prostate cancer patients submitted to radical prostatectomy) (Table 1).

Table 1. Clinical and histopathological characteristics of patients with bladder carcinoma (BlCa), normal bladder mucosae (NB), healthy donors (HD) and inflammatory controls (IC).

Clinicopaphological Features	Tissues		Urines				
			Testing Set		Validation Sets		
	Bladder UC	Normal Bladder Mucosae	Bladder UC	Healthy Donors	Bladder UC	Healthy Donors (#1)	Inflammatory Controls (#2)
Patients, n	94	19	27	24	100	57	174
Gender, n							
Males	78	19	20	13	79	16	132
Females	16	0	7	12	21	41	42
Median age, yrs	69	63	69	45	68	49	64
(range)	(45–91)	(48–75)	(47–88)	(39–61)	(38–91)	(41–64)	(18–92)
Grade, n							
Papillary, low-grade	34	n.a.	13	n.a.	51	n.a.	n.a.
Papillary, high-grade	33	n.a.	8	n.a.	26	n.a.	n.a.
Invasive, high-grade	27	n.a.	6	n.a.	23	n.a.	n.a.
Invasion of Muscular Layer, n							
NMIBC	67	n.a.	19	n.a.	77	n.a.	n.a.
MIBC	27	n.a.	8	n.a.	23	n.a.	n.a.

#1—Validation Set #1; #2—Validation Set #2; yrs—years; n.a.—non applicable; NMIBC—Non-Muscle Invasive Bladder Cancer; MIBC—Muscle Invasive Bladder Cancer, UC—Urothelial Carcinoma.

2.2. Urine Sample Collection and Processing

For the "Testing sets", 27 voided urine samples (one per patient) were collected from BlCa patients, diagnosed and treated between 2006 and 2016 at IPO Porto, as well as a set of 24 voided urine samples from healthy donors (HD), also from IPO Porto, with no personal or familial history of cancer, used as controls (Table 1). The "Validation sets" comprised: (1) 100 urine samples from BlCa patients, diagnosed and treated between 2002 and 2016 at IPO Porto, and 57 urine samples from HD collected at IPO Porto, and (2) an independent set of control urine sediments ($n = 174$) from patients diagnosed with urinary tract inflammatory conditions (IC), diagnosed between 2008 and 2014 at the University Hospital of Cordoba (UHC). All BlCa patients' urines were obtained before treatment Moreover, all sets of samples were collected from different cohorts of patients. Informed consent was obtained from patients and controls after approval from the ethics committees of IPO Porto and UHC (CES-IPO 019/08, approval date: 16th January 2008). All urine samples were processed by immediate centrifugation at 4000 rpm for 10 min; the respective pellet was washed twice with phosphate-buffered saline (PBS) and stored at −80 °C.

2.3. Nucleic Acids Isolation, Bisulfite Modification and Multiplex qMSP Analysis

DNA was extracted from frozen BlCa and NB tissues, and all urine sample sets, using a standard phenol-chloroform protocol [16], and its concentration determined using a Qubit 3 Fluorometer (Thermo Fisher Scientific, Waltham, MA, USA). Bisulfite modification was performed through sodium bisulfite, using the EZ DNA Methylation-Gold™ Kit (Zymo Research, Irvine, CA, USA), according to manufacturer's protocol. For this, 1000 ng and 50 ng of DNA were converted for tissues and urine sediments, respectively. Quantitative methylation levels were performed using Xpert Fast Probe Master Mix (GRiSP, Porto, Portugal), and multiplex reactions were run in triplicates in 96-well plates using an Applied Biosystems 7500 Sequence Detector (Perkin Elmer, Waltham, CA, USA), with Beta-Actin (ACTB) as internal reference gene for normalization. Primer and probe sequences were designed using Methyl Primer Express 1.0 and purchased from Sigma-Aldrich (St. Louis, MO, USA) (Supplementary Table S1). Additionally, six serial dilutions (dilution factor of 5×) of a fully methylated bisulphite modified universal DNA control were included in each plate to generate a standard curve. In each sample and for each gene, the relative DNA methylation levels were determined using the following formula: ((target gene/ACTB) ×1000). A run was considered valid when previously reported criteria were met [11].

2.4. Statistical Analysis

Differences in quantitative methylation values were assessed with the non-parametric Mann-Whitney U (MW) and Kruskal-Wallis (KW) tests. Associations between age, gender, grade, invasion of muscular layer and methylation levels were carried out using Spearman's correlation, MW or KW tests, as appropriate. For multiple comparisons, Bonferroni's correction was applied in pairwise comparisons.

Biomarker performance parameters, including sensitivity, specificity, positive predictive value (PPV), negative predictive value (NPV), accuracy and positive and negative likelihood ratios (LR), were estimated [17]. Receiver operator characteristics (ROC) curves were constructed by plotting the true positive (sensitivity) against false positive (1-specificity) rate, and the area under the curve (AUC) was calculated. The higher value obtained from the sum of sensitivity and 1-specificity in each ROC-curve was used as cut-off to categorise samples as methylated or non-methylated. ROC curves were constructed using logistic regression model for DNA methylation panel. Disease-specific and disease-free survival curves (Kaplan-Meier with log rank test) were computed for standard variables and for categorised genes' promoter methylation status. A Cox-regression model comprising all significant variables (univariable and multivariable model) was computed to assess the relative contribution of each variable to the follow-up status. All two-tailed p values were derived from statistical tests, using a computer-assisted program (SPSS Version 26.0, IBM, Armonk, NY, EUA) and the results were considered statistically significant at $p < 0.05$. Bonferroni's correction for multiple comparisons was used when applicable.

3. Results

3.1. Methylation Analysis and Performance of the Multiplex Panel in BlCa Tissue Series

To confirm the previously published performance of $miR663a$ and VIM promoter methylation as BlCa biomarkers, tissue samples were tested. As expected, both $miR663a$ and VIM were found hypermethylated (76.6% and 94.4%, respectively) in most BlCa tissue samples, and methylation levels were significantly higher compared to NB ($p < 0.0001$ and $p < 0.0001$, respectively) (Figure 1A). The two genes independently performed well as BlCa detection biomarkers in tissues, with an AUC of 0.979 for VIM_{me} (95% confidence interval (CI): 0.956–1.002, $p < 0.0001$), and of 0.897 for $miR663a_{me}$ (95% CI: 0.836–0.959, $p < 0.0001$). Moreover, in combination as multiplex panel, it accurately discriminated BlCa from NB with 96.3% sensitivity and 88.2% specificity, corresponding to an AUC of 0.982 (Figure 1B; Supplementary Table S2).

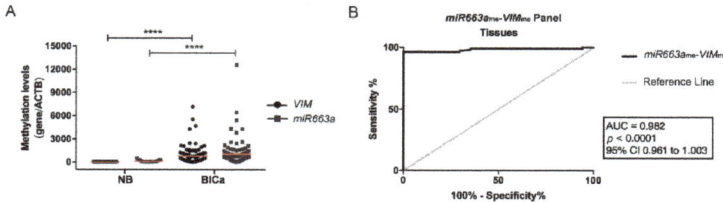

Figure 1. (**A**) Distribution of VIM_{me} and $miR663a_{me}$ levels in normal bladder mucosae (NB; $n = 19$) and bladder carcinoma (BlCa; $n = 94$) tissue samples. Mann-Whitney U test, **** $p < 0.0001$. Median is represented by the red line. (**B**) Receiver operator characteristic (ROC) curve evaluating the performance of the VIM_{me}-$miR663a_{me}$ panel for the identification of BlCa in tissue samples. (AUC—Area under the curve; CI—Confidence interval; ACTB—Beta-Actin; VIM—Vimentin).

3.2. Methylation Analysis and Performance of Multiplex Panel in BlCa Testing Set

Paralleling the previous observations in tissues, $miR663a_{me}$ and VIM_{me} levels were significantly higher in BlCa urine samples than in those of controls ($p < 0.0001$ and $p < 0.0001$, Figure 2A), and the multiplex panel discriminated BlCa from HD with 92.6% sensitivity and 90% NPV (Supplementary Table S2), corresponding to an AUC of 0.83 (Figure 2B).

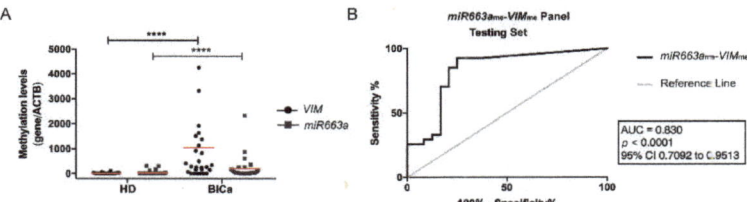

Figure 2. (**A**) Distribution of VIM_{me} and $miR663a_{me}$ levels in the Testing Cohort, composed by healthy donors (HD; $n = 24$) and bladder carcinoma (BlCa; $n = 27$) urine samples. Mann-Whitney U test, **** $p < 0.0001$. Median is represented by the red line. (**B**) Receiver operator characteristic (ROC) curve evaluating the performance of the VIM_{me}-$miR663a_{me}$ panel for the identification of BlCa in urine samples of the Testing Cohort. (AUC—Area under the curve; CI—Confidence interval; ACTB—Beta-Actin; VIM—Vimentin).

3.3. Methylation Analysis and Performance of VIM_{me} and $miR663_{me}$ Multiplex Panel for BlCa vs. HD

In line with the testing set results, a higher number of malignant samples disclosed significantly higher VIM_{me} and $miR663_{me}$ levels than HDs ($p < 0.0001$ and $p < 0.0001$, respectively) in the validation sets (Figure 3A). ROC curve analysis confirmed a high discriminative ability of VIM_{me}-$miR663_{me}$ panel, with an AUC of 0.91 (Figure 3B). Indeed, the multiplex panel discriminated BlCa from HD subjects with 87% sensitivity and 86% specificity (Table 2).

Table 2. Performance of VIM_{me}-$miR663a_{me}$ panel for the detection of bladder cancer in Validation Cohorts #1 and #2. (PPV—positive predictive value; NPV—negative predictive value).

Samples	Biomarker Performance	$miR663a_{me}$-VIM_{me} (%)
Validation #1	Sensitivity	87.0
	Specificity	86.0
	PPV	91.6
	NPV	79.0
	Accuracy	86.6
Validation #2	Sensitivity	80.0
	Specificity	75.3
	PPV	65.0
	NPV	86.8
	Accuracy	77.0

PPV—Positive Predictive Value; NPV—Negative Predictive Value.

Remarkably, the proportion of true positive cases detected by the VIM_{me}-$miR663_{me}$ multiplex panel was significantly higher than that of urine cytology ($p < 0.001$). Indeed, of 46 BlCa cases with valid urine cytology results, only 19 were classified as positive, 17 as negative and 10 as "inconclusive/suspicious", corresponding to 41% sensitivity (Figure 4). Contrarily, the VIM_{me}-$miR663_{me}$ multiplex panel correctly identified 40/46 cases as BlCa, corresponding to an overall sensitivity of 87% (Figure 4). Importantly, 12 of 14 low-grade papillary carcinomas were accurately identified by VIM_{me}-$miR663_{me}$ multiplex panel, whereas cytology merely identified four cases.

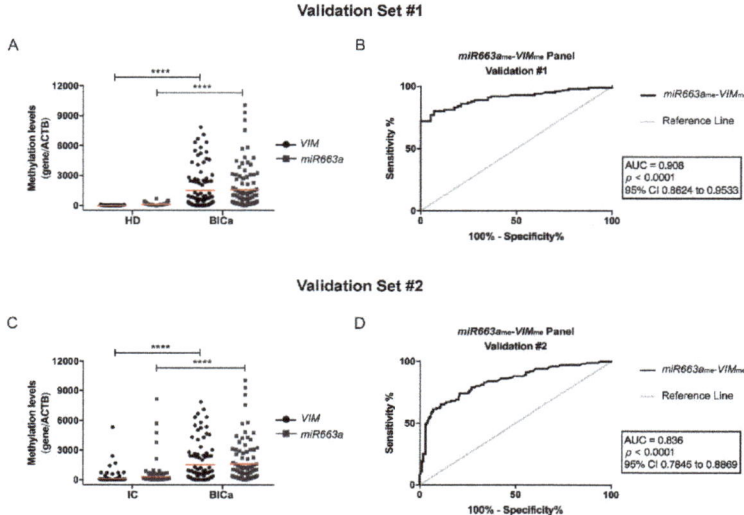

Figure 3. (**A**) Distribution of VIM_{me} and $miR663a_{me}$ levels in the Validation Cohort #1, composed by healthy donors (HD; $n = 57$) and bladder carcinoma (BlCa; $n = 100$) urine samples. Mann-Whitney U (MW) test, **** $p < 0.0001$. Median is represented by the red line. (**B**) Receiver operator characteristic (ROC) curve evaluating the performance of the VIM_{me}-$miR663a_{me}$ panel for the identification of BlCa in urine samples of the Validation Cohort #1. (**C**) Distribution of VIM_{me} and $miR663a_{me}$ levels in the Validation Cohort #2, composed by inflammatory controls (IC; $n = 174$) and bladder carcinoma (BlCa; $n = 100$) urine samples. MW test, **** $p < 0.0001$. (**D**) ROC curve evaluating the performance of the VIM_{me}-$miR663a_{me}$ panel for the identification of BlCa in urine samples of the Validation Cohort #2. (AUC—Area under the curve; CI—Confidence interval; ACTB—Beta-Actin; VIM—Vimentin).

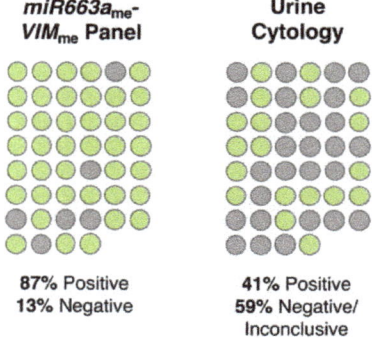

Figure 4. Representation of the percentage of bladder cancer (BlCa) cases correctly identified with the VIM_{me}-$miR663a_{me}$ panel and a standard urine cytology analysis. Green circles represent positive cases, grey circles represent negative/inconclusive cases.

3.4. Methylation Analysis and Performance of VIM_{me} and $miR663_{me}$ Multiplex Panel for BlCa vs. IC

In urine samples, VIM_{me}-$miR663_{me}$ levels discriminated BlCa from IC patients (Figure 3C), with 80% sensitivity, 75.3% specificity and, importantly, 86.8% NPV (Table 2), corresponding to an AUC of 0.836 (Figure 3D). Remarkably, a 2.86 Positive LR and a Negative LR of 0.21 were also disclosed by VIM_{me}-$miR663_{me}$ multiplex panel in this setting.

3.5. Clinicopathologic Correlations and Survival Analyses

High-grade papillary BlCa showed significantly higher $miR663a_{me}$ levels than low-grade papillary BlCa ($p = 0.007$), in tissue samples. The same was observed in urine samples from the validation set ($p = 0.0072$), a result which was extensive to VIM_{me} ($p = 0.0052$) (Supplementary Figure S1). No additional associations were disclosed between VIM_{me} and $miR663a_{me}$ levels and other standard clinical variables, including patients' age and gender.

Follow-up data was available for 91 (out of 94) IPO Porto's BlCa patients that provided tissue samples. The median follow-up time was 66 months (range: 1–203 months). At the last follow-up timepoint, 30 patients were alive with no evidence of cancer, 12 patients were alive with disease, 29 had deceased due to BlCa and 23 died from other causes. Univariable and multivariable Cox regression analysis were performed, including the variables grade, invasion of muscular layer, gender and age. As expected, a poor outcome was depicted for patients with higher grade and muscle invasive BlCa ($p = 0.001$ and $p < 0.0001$, respectively) (Table 3). In the multivariate model for disease-specific survival, $miR663a_{me}$ levels, higher grade and muscle invasion were independent predictors of outcome ($p = 0.04$, $p = 0.035$ and $p = 0.031$, respectively; Table 3). Moreover, after categorization into NMIBC vs. MIBC, tumours with higher $miR663a_{me}$ levels implied a 3.7-fold increased risk of cancer-related death among patients with MIBC (95% CI: 1.32–10.25, $p = 0.013$; Supplementary Figure S2). Contrarily, no associations were found for $miR663a_{me}$ or VIM_{me} levels concerning disease-free survival.

Table 3. Cox regression models assessing the potential of clinical and VIMme and miR663ame levels in the prediction of disease-specific survival for bladder carcinoma (BlCa) patients.

Disease-specific Survival	Variables	Hazard Ratio (HR)	95% CI for OR	p
Univariate	Invasion of muscular layer	6.15	2.76–13.72	0.0001
	Grade			
	PLG vs. PHG	15.59	2.03–119.94	0.008
	PLG vs. IHG	32.83	4.31–250.06	0.001
	Age	2.34	0.98–5.59	0.060
	Gender	1.02	0.39–2.70	0.970
	miR663a methylation ≤ median	1.61	0.75–3.48	0.225
	VIM methylation ≤ median	1.07	0.50–2.28	0.861
Multivariate	Invasion of muscular layer	3.54	1.12–11.19	0.031
	Grade			
	PLG vs. PHG	8.03	0.97–66.32	0.053
	PLG vs. IHG	11.89	1.18–119.37	0.035
	miR663a methylation ≤ median	2.67	1.05–6.81	0.040
	VIM methylation ≤ median	1.12	0.51–2.42	0.783

CI—confidence interval; OR—odds ratio; PLG—papillary low-grade; PHG—papillary high-grade; IHG—invasive high-grade.

4. Discussion

Bladder cancer is a major health concern worldwide, with an expected significant increase in incidence and mortality within the next two decades [1,2]. Early detection is critical for adequate management, aiming to reduce disease-specific mortality, as well as the economic burden imposed by BlCa treatment and follow-up. Because currently available diagnostic tools require invasive examination [13,14], development of non-invasive and less costly tests for early detection and monitoring are likely to have a significant impact in clinical practice. Although several molecular biomarkers, including epigenetic-based, have been developed for that end, discrimination of BlCa from other urinary tract malignancies and, more importantly, from benign conditions causing haematuria, including inflammatory diseases, remains a challenge. Indeed, most control samples used in biomarker discovery studies, including our own, mostly comprise normal/healthy donors, disregarding the fact that a biomarker-based test would be offered to an "at-risk" population, including patients experiencing suspicious symptoms. Therefore, based on two previously published studies by our research team [11,12], we tested whether a $miR663a_{me}$ and VIM_{me} multiplex panel could accurately discriminate BlCa from normal individuals and those afflicted with inflammatory conditions of the genitourinary tract.

Because both $miR663a_{me}$ and VIM_{me} were previously assessed using two different "simplex" multi-gene biomarker panels, we firstly tested $miR663a_{me}$ and VIM_{me} in multiplex in a consecutive series of primary BlCa tissue samples and normal urothelial mucosae to confirm those previous results. Indeed, employing a multiplex reaction allows for downscaling the initial tissue/body fluid sample requirements, but also the quantity of DNA required for each test [18]. Remarkably, as expected, the $miR663a_{me}$-VIM_{me} multiplex panel discriminated BlCa from NB tissues with high sensitivity and specificity (96.3% and 88.2%, respectively), confirming the previous observations for the two markers separately [11,12]. In urine samples from the testing set, although the performance of the multiplex panel was slightly inferior to that of tissues, 92.6% sensitivity and 90% NPV was reached. Indeed, it should be recalled that a relatively small number of cancer cells are exfoliated into urine, which are subsequently "diluted" among a larger population of normal-looking urothelial cells. Thus, the tumour DNA content in urine is actually minute [19] and sensitivity over 90% should be regarded as a very encouraging result. Furthermore, in the validation set, comprising a larger independent cohort, specificity of the $miR663a_{me}$-VIM_{me} multiplex panel increased to 86%, further increasing the potential usefulness of the test.

It should be emphasised, however, that the foremost aim of this study was to assess the multiplex panel ability to discriminate BlCa from IC, since this panel is envisaged to be tested in an "at-risk" population, including individuals complaining of haematuria, many of which will be found to harbour urinary tract inflammatory conditions. Although, in this setting, sensitivity and specificity were slightly reduced, NPV increased (86.8%), which is an important finding [20]. Indeed, it is expected that among tested individuals, most will not have a neoplastic condition and, thus, the higher the NPV, the larger the proportion of those subjects that will not be submitted to confirmatory, invasive, procedures, supporting the good performance of the test in discriminating patients negative for malignant condition. Importantly, an LR (+) of 2.86 and an LR (−) of 0.21 values were observed, indicating that a negative result decreases by 30% the probability of misdiagnosis [17].

Despite the fact that several studies suggest various genomic mutations and/or proteins' expression deregulation as biomarkers for BlCa detection and prognostication [21], the search for novel epigenetic biomarkers, mostly DNA methylation-based, for BlCa detection has been attempted by several research teams, probably due to the stability of the markers and the possibility of high-throughput tests. Although some of those previous studies report an apparently superior performance to the panel reported herein, it should be recalled that in most cases the patients' series were smaller, only healthy donors were included as controls or these were comprised of a mixed group of healthy donors and patients with diverse urological diseases, and/or did not use a multiplex approach, which might impact in sample availability, testing time length and cost [22–28]. Roperch et al. proposed a three gene multiplex methylation panel (*HS3ST2*, *SEPTIN9* and *SLIT2*) combined with *FGFR3* mutations assessment, age and smoking-status at time of diagnosis in a multivariate model, for diagnosis of NMIBC in urine samples, disclosing 97.6% sensitivity and 84.8% specificity, in a smaller control cohort [29]. Nonetheless, this strategy might be more difficult to implement in clinical practice, since it requires both mutation and methylation analyses, in which the multiplex is performed in two distinct gene duplex reactions. Similarly, Dahmcke et al. proposed a six gene methylation panel (*SALL3*, *ONECUT2*, *CCNA1*, *BCL2*, *EOMES* and *VIM*) combined with the mutational analysis of *TERT* and *FGFR3*, for early detection of BlCa, in urine samples, comparing BlCa patients and patients with gross haematuria [30]. Although this panel disclosed higher sensitivity (97%), specificity was similar (76.9%) [30], and, once again, our test uses a single technique in a single reaction, requiring less amount of sample, enabling shorter response time, reduced technical skills and lower cost.

Although urine cytology and UroVysion™ fluorescence in situ hybridization (FISH) assay are the two most commonly used urine-based tests in daily practice, they present important limitations. On one hand, UroVysion™ presents a not-negligible rate of false positive results; on the other hand, urine cytology has limited accuracy, especially in low grade tumours detection [6,31,32]. Although no direct comparison can be done with UroVysion^{TM}, the 91.6% PPV obtained for the multiplex panel clearly demonstrates higher accuracy in identifying true positive BlCa cases. In the present study, urine cytology reached 41% sensitivity, which was easily surpassed by the 86% displayed by $miR663a_{me}$-VIM_{me} multiplex panel. Notwithstanding, urine cytology remains an easy-to-perform and informative test, as it allows pathologists to have the first look at exfoliated neoplastic cells in urine. Having that in mind, we propose an algorithm where a urine cytology and the $miR563a_{me}$-VIM_{me} multiplex panel could be combined as first-line diagnostic tests in patients with common urinary complaints, with the ultimate goal of reducing the number of unnecessary cystoscopies, which are invasive, uncomfortable and costly procedures (Figure 5).

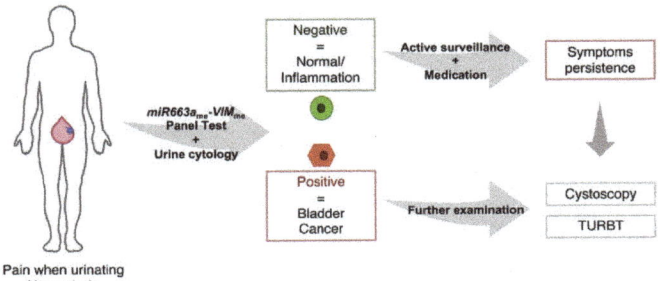

Figure 5. Proposed algorithm for the combination of urine cytology and VIM_{me}-$miR663a_{me}$ panel as a first-line diagnostic tests in patients with common urinary complaints. (TURBT—Transurethral Resection of Bladder Tumour).

In this work, we further explored the prognostic ability of the gene methylation markers, aiming to strengthen its clinical potential. Interestingly, survival analysis revealed that high $miR663a_{me}$ levels independently predicted poor disease-specific survival in BlCa patients, especially those with MIBC. Thus, the $miR663a_{me}$-VIM_{me} multiplex panel not only conveys diagnostic, but also prognostic information.

Taking into account the promising results obtained, unveiling the putative biological relevance of $miR663a$ and VIM promoter methylation in bladder carcinogenesis may provide new important insights. VIM encodes for vimentin, an intermediate filament characteristic of cells with mesenchymal phenotype, not expressed in most normal epithelia (including urothelium), nor in most carcinomas [33]. VIM de-novo expression or overexpression has been reported in various epithelial cancers, including those of prostate [34], breast [35] and lung [36], associating with increased tumour growth and invasion. In these instances, vimentin expression has been associated with epithelial to mesenchymal transition (EMT), a biological process associated with tumour invasiveness [33]. Although VIM promoter methylation has been proposed as a detection and/or prognostic marker for other malignancies, biological functions are yet to be truly explored. Moreover, microRNAs have been extensively implicated in urological malignancies [37]. Interestingly, a dual role has already been described for miR663a, having a tumour suppressive activity in thyroid carcinoma [38] and glioblastoma [39], whereas an oncogenic function was reported in prostate cancer [40] and osteosarcoma [41]. Additionally, miR663a's downregulation fostered cell proliferation by JunD overexpression in small-cell lung carcinoma [42], and HMGA2 in hepatocellular carcinoma [43], while Transforming Growth Factor-1 (TGF-β1) [44] overexpression was linked with invasion in the tumour type. Nevertheless, it should be recalled that not all biomarkers require to have a relevant biological role in tumorigenesis.

Importantly, to assure accuracy and validity of the proposed methylation multiplex test, additional validation by others, with larger sets of samples from prospectively collected data (from both BlCa and inflammatory conditions) is warrant.

5. Conclusions

In summary, we demonstrated that a $miR663a_{me}$-VIM_{me} multiplex panel accurately identifies BlCa, allowing for precise identification of this common neoplasm in urine samples. Importantly, it also discriminates BlCa patients from those with urinary tract inflammatory conditions, although with inferior performance comparatively to healthy subjects. Thus, the implementation of this panel might assist clinicians in better stratifying patients for confirmatory, invasive examinations, ultimately improving the cost-effectiveness of BlCa diagnosis and management. Moreover, in the same analysis, $miR663a_{me}$ analysis would identify patients at higher risk for cancer progression, further highlighting the promise of this panel for patient monitoring.

Supplementary Materials: The following are available online at http://www.mdpi.com/2077-0383/9/2/605/s1, Figure S1: Distribution of $miR663a_{me}$ and VIM_{me} levels in bladder carcinoma tissue samples categorised by grade; Figure S2: Kaplan-Meyer curves representing disease-specific survival according to $miR663a_{me}$ status; Table S1: Sequences of the primers and probes used in the quantitative methylation-specific PCR experiments; Table S2: Performance of VIM_{me}, $miR663a_{me}$ and VIM_{me}-$miR663a_{me}$ panel for the detection of bladder cancer in Tissues and Testing Set.

Author Contributions: Conceptualization, S.M.-R., R.H. and C.J.; methodology, S.M.-R., A.B., J.T.-M., I.C., D.M., P.M. and J.O.; formal analysis, S.M.-R. and L.A.; writing—original draft preparation, S.M.-R.; review and editing, R.H., C.J. and A.L.-B.; supervision, R.H. and C.J. All authors have read and agreed to the published version of the manuscript.

Funding: This research was funded by the Research Center of Portuguese Institute of Porto (CI-IPOP-27-2016). S.M-R. was supported by the FCT—Fundação para a Ciência e Tecnologia Grant (SFRH/BD/112673/2015).

Acknowledgments: The authors are grateful to the patients that volunteered to provide samples and to all the personnel of the Departments of Pathology (section of Cytopathology) and of Urology of Portuguese Oncology Institute of Porto that kindly collaborated in this study.

Conflicts of Interest: The authors declare no conflict of interest. The funders had no role in the design of the study; in the collection, analyses or interpretation of data; in the writing of the manuscript, or in the decision to publish the results.

References

1. Ferlay, J.; Ervik, M.; Lam, F.; Colombet, M.; Mery, L.; Piñeros, M.; Znaor, A.; Soerjomataram, I.; Bray, F. Global Cancer Observatory: Cancer Tomorrow. Available online: https://gco.iarc.fr/tomorrow/home (accessed on 26 October 2019).
2. Antoni, S.; Ferlay, J.; Soerjomataram, I.; Znaor, A.; Jemal, A.; Bray, F. Bladder Cancer Incidence and Mortality: A Global Overview and Recent Trends. *Eur. Urol.* **2017**, *71*, 96–108. [CrossRef]
3. Sanli, O.; Dobruch, J.; Knowles, M.A.; Burger, M.; Alemozaffar, M.; Nielsen, M.E.; Lotan, Y. Bladder cancer. *Nat. Rev. Dis. Primers* **2017**, *3*, 17022. [CrossRef]
4. International Agency for Cancer Research. *WHO Classification of Tumours of the Urinary System and Male Genital Organs*, 4th ed.; Moch, H., Ulbright, T., Humphrey, P., Reuter, V., Eds.; IARC: Lyon, France, 2016.
5. Kaufman, D.S.; Shipley, W.U.; Feldman, A.S. Bladder cancer. *Lancet (London, England)* **2009**, *374*, 239–249. [CrossRef]
6. Babjuk, M.; Burger, M.; Comperat, E.M.; Gontero, P.; Mostafid, A.H.; Palou, J.; van Rhijn, B.W.G.; Roupret, M.; Shariat, S.F.; Sylvester, R.; et al. European Association of Urology Guidelines on Non-muscle-invasive Bladder Cancer (TaT1 and Carcinoma In Situ)—2019 Update. *Eur. Urol.* **2019**, *76*, 639–657. [CrossRef]
7. Alfred Witjes, J.; Lebret, T.; Comperat, E.M.; Cowan, N.C.; De Santis, M.; Bruins, H.M.; Hernandez, V.; Espinos, E.L.; Dunn, J.; Rouanne, M.; et al. Updated 2016 EAU Guidelines on Muscle-invasive and Metastatic Bladder Cancer. *Eur. Urol.* **2017**, *71*, 462–475. [CrossRef]
8. Leal, J.; Luengo-Fernandez, R.; Sullivan, R.; Witjes, J.A. Economic Burden of Bladder Cancer Across the European Union. *Eur. Urol.* **2016**, *69*, 438–447. [CrossRef]
9. Esteller, M. Epigenetics in cancer. *N. Engl. J. Med.* **2008**, *358*, 1148–1159. [CrossRef] [PubMed]
10. Costa-Pinheiro, P.; Montezuma, D.; Henrique, R.; Jeronimo, C. Diagnostic and prognostic epigenetic biomarkers in cancer. *Epigenomics* **2015**, *7*, 1003–1015. [CrossRef] [PubMed]

11. Costa, V.L.; Henrique, R.; Danielsen, S.A.; Duarte-Pereira, S.; Eknaes, M.; Skotheim, R.I.; Rodrigues, A.; Magalhaes, J.S.; Oliveira, J.; Lothe, R.A.; et al. Three epigenetic biomarkers, GDF15, TMEFF2, and VIM, accurately predict bladder cancer from DNA-based analyses of urine samples. *Clin. Cancer Res.* **2010**, *16*, 5842–5851. [CrossRef] [PubMed]
12. Padrao, N.A.; Monteiro-Reis, S.; Torres-Ferreira, J.; Antunes, L.; Leca, L.; Montezuma, D.; Ramalho-Carvalho, J.; Dias, P.C.; Monteiro, P.; Oliveira, J.; et al. MicroRNA promoter methylation: A new tool for accurate detection of urothelial carcinoma. *Br. J. Cancer* **2017**, *116*, 634–639. [CrossRef]
13. Heller, M.T.; Tublin, M.E. In search of a consensus: Evaluation of the patient with hematuria in an era of cost containment. *Am. J. Roentgenol.* **2014**, *202*, 1179–1186. [CrossRef] [PubMed]
14. Grover, S.; Srivastava, A.; Lee, R.; Tewari, A.K.; Te, A.E. Role of inflammation in bladder function and interstitial cystitis. *Ther. Adv. Urol.* **2011**, *3*, 19–33. [CrossRef] [PubMed]
15. Humphrey, P.A.; Moch, H.; Cubilla, A.L.; Ulbright, T.M.; Reuter, V.E. The 2016 WHO Classification of Tumours of the Urinary System and Male Genital Organs-Part B: Prostate and Bladder Tumours. *Eur. Urol.* **2016**, *70*, 106–119. [CrossRef] [PubMed]
16. Pearson, H.; Stirling, D. DNA extraction from tissue. In *PCR Protocols*, 2nd ed.; Bartlett, J.M.S., Stirling, D., Eds.; Humana Press: Totowa, NJ, USA, 2003.
17. McGee, S. Simplifying likelihood ratios. *J. Gen. Intern. Med.* **2002**, *17*, 646–649. [CrossRef]
18. Guest, P.C. Multiplex Biomarker Approaches to Enable Point-of-Care Testing and Personalized Medicine. *Methods Mol. Biol.* **2017**, *1546*, 311–315. [CrossRef]
19. Larsen, L.K.; Lind, G.E.; Guldberg, P.; Dahl, C. DNA-Methylation-Based Detection of Urological Cancer in Urine: Overview of Biomarkers and Considerations on Biomarker Design, Source of DNA, and Detection Technologies. *Int. J. Mol. Sci.* **2019**, *20*, 2657. [CrossRef]
20. Anna K Füzéry, D.W.C. Cancer Biomarker Assays: Performance Standards. In *Biomarkers in Cancer Screening and Early Detection*, 1st ed.; Srivastava, S., Ed.; John Wiley & Sons: Hoboken, NJ, USA, 2017; pp. 267–276.
21. Tan, W.S.; Tan, W.P.; Tan, M.Y.; Khetrapal, P.; Dong, L.; de Winter, P.; Feber, A.; Kelly, J.D. Novel urinary biomarkers for the detection of bladder cancer: A systematic review. *Cancer Treat. Rev.* **2018**, *69*, 39–52. [CrossRef]
22. Chihara, Y.; Kanai, Y.; Fujimoto, H.; Sugano, K.; Kawashima, K.; Liang, G.; Jones, P.A.; Fujimoto, K.; Kuniyasu, H.; Hirao, Y. Diagnostic markers of urothelial cancer based on DNA methylation analysis. *BMC Cancer* **2013**, *13*, 275. [CrossRef]
23. Wang, Y.; Yu, Y.; Ye, R.; Zhang, D.; Li, Q.; An, D.; Fang, L.; Lin, Y.; Hou, Y.; Xu, A.; et al. An epigenetic biomarker combination of PCDH17 and POU4F2 detects bladder cancer accurately by methylation analyses of urine sediment DNA in Han Chinese. *Oncotarget* **2016**, *7*, 2754–2764. [CrossRef]
24. Yegin, Z.; Gunes, S.; Buyukalpelli, R. Hypermethylation of TWIST1 and NID2 in tumor tissues and voided urine in urinary bladder cancer patients. *DNA Cell Biol.* **2013**, *32*, 386–392. [CrossRef]
25. Renard, I.; Joniau, S.; van Cleynenbreugel, B.; Collette, C.; Naome, C.; Vlassenbroeck, I.; Nicolas, H.; de Leval, J.; Straub, J.; Van Criekinge, W.; et al. Identification and validation of the methylated TWIST1 and NID2 genes through real-time methylation-specific polymerase chain reaction assays for the noninvasive detection of primary bladder cancer in urine samples. *Eur. Urol.* **2010**, *58*, 96–104. [CrossRef] [PubMed]
26. Yu, J.; Zhu, T.; Wang, Z.; Zhang, H.; Qian, Z.; Xu, H.; Gao, B.; Wang, W.; Gu, L.; Meng, J.; et al. A novel set of DNA methylation markers in urine sediments for sensitive/specific detection of bladder cancer. *Clin. Cancer Res.* **2007**, *13*, 7296–7304. [CrossRef] [PubMed]
27. Sun, J.; Chen, Z.; Zhu, T.; Yu, J.; Ma, K.; Zhang, H.; He, Y.; Luo, X.; Zhu, J. Hypermethylated SFRP1, but none of other nine genes "informative" for western countries, is valuable for bladder cancer detection in Mainland China. *J. Cancer Res. Clin. Oncol.* **2009**, *135*, 1717–1727. [CrossRef]
28. Chan, M.W.; Chan, L.W.; Tang, N.L.; Tong, J.H.; Lo, K.W.; Lee, T.L.; Cheung, H.Y.; Wong, W.S.; Chan, P.S.; Lai, F.M.; et al. Hypermethylation of multiple genes in tumor tissues and voided urine in urinary bladder cancer patients. *Clin. Cancer Res.* **2002**, *8*, 464–470. [PubMed]
29. Roperch, J.P.; Grandchamp, B.; Desgrandchamps, F.; Mongiat-Artus, P.; Ravery, V.; Ouzaid, I.; Roupret, M.; Phe, V.; Ciofu, C.; Tubach, F.; et al. Promoter hypermethylation of HS3ST2, SEPTIN9 and SLIT2 combined with FGFR3 mutations as a sensitive/specific urinary assay for diagnosis and surveillance in patients with low or high-risk non-muscle-invasive bladder cancer. *BMC Cancer* **2016**, *16*, 704. [CrossRef]

30. Dahmcke, C.M.; Steven, K.E.; Larsen, L.K.; Poulsen, A.L.; Abdul-Al, A.; Dahl, C.; Guldberg, P. A Prospective Blinded Evaluation of Urine-DNA Testing for Detection of Urothelial Bladder Carcinoma in Patients with Gross Hematuria. *Eur. Urol.* **2016**, *70*, 916–919. [CrossRef]
31. Brimo, F.; Vollmer, R.T.; Case, B.; Aprikian, A.; Kassouf, W.; Auger, M. Accuracy of urine cytology and the significance of an atypical category. *Am. J. Clin. Pathol.* **2009**, *132*, 785–793. [CrossRef]
32. Lavery, H.J.; Zaharieva, B.; McFaddin, A.; Heerema, N.; Pohar, K.S. A prospective comparison of UroVysion FISH and urine cytology in bladder cancer detection. *BMC Cancer* **2017**, *17*, 247. [CrossRef]
33. Satelli, A.; Li, S. Vimentin in cancer and its potential as a molecular target for cancer therapy. *Cell Mol. Life Sci.* **2011**, *68*, 3033. [CrossRef]
34. Singh, S.; Sadacharan, S.; Su, S.; Belldegrun, A.; Persad, S.; Singh, G. Overexpression of vimentin: Role in the invasive phenotype in an androgen-independent model of prostate cancer. *Cancer Res.* **2003**, *63*, 2306–2311.
35. Kokkinos, M.I.; Wafai, R.; Wong, M.K.; Newgreen, D.F.; Thompson, E.W.; Waltham, M. Vimentin and Epithelial-Mesenchymal Transition in Human Breast Cancer—Observations in vitro and in vivo. *Cells Tissues Organs* **2007**, *185*, 191–203. [CrossRef] [PubMed]
36. Al-Saad, S.; Al-Shibli, K.; Donnem, T.; Persson, M.; Bremnes, R.M.; Busund, L.T. The prognostic impact of NF-kappaB p105, vimentin, E-cadherin and Par6 expression in epithelial and stromal compartment in non-small-cell lung cancer. *Br. J. Cancer* **2008**, *99*, 1476–1483. [CrossRef] [PubMed]
37. Jerónimo, C.; Henrique, R. Epigenetic biomarkers in urological tumors: A systematic review. *Cancer Lett.* **2014**, *342*, 264–274. [CrossRef] [PubMed]
38. Wang, Z.; Zhang, H.; Zhang, P.; Dong, W.; He, L. MicroRNA-663 suppresses cell invasion and migration by targeting transforming growth factor beta 1 in papillary thyroid carcinoma. *Tumour Biol.* **2015**, *37*, 7633–7644. [CrossRef]
39. Shi, Y.; Chen, C.; Yu, S.; Liu, Q.; Rao, J.; Zhang, H.R.; Xiao, H.L.; Fu, T.W.; Long, H.; He, Z.; et al. MiR-663 suppresses oncogenic function of CXCR4 in glioblastoma. *Clin. Cancer Res.* **2015**, *21*, 4004–4013. [CrossRef]
40. Jiao, L.; Deng, Z.; Xu, C.; Yu, Y.; Li, Y.; Yang, C.; Chen, J.; Liu, Z.; Huang, G.; Li, L.C.; et al. MiR-663 induces castration-resistant prostate cancer transformation and predicts clinical recurrence. *J. Cell Physiol.* **2014**, *229*, 834–844. [CrossRef]
41. Huang, C.; Sun, Y.; Ma, S.; Vadamootoo, A.S.; Wang, L.; Jin, C. Identification of circulating miR-663a as a potential biomarker for diagnosing osteosarcoma. *Pathol. Res. Pract.* **2019**, *215*, 152411. [CrossRef]
42. Zhang, Y.; Xu, X.; Zhang, M.; Wang, X.; Bai, X.; Li, H.; Kan, L.; Zhou, Y.; Niu, H.; He, P. MicroRNA-663a is downregulated in non-small cell lung cancer and inhibits proliferation and invasion by targeting JunD. *BMC Cancer* **2016**, *16*, 315. [CrossRef]
43. Huang, W.; Li, J.; Guo, X.; Zhao, Y.; Yuan, X. MiR-663a inhibits hepatocellular carcinoma cell proliferation and invasion by targeting HMGA2. *Biomed. Pharmacother.* **2016**, *81*, 431–438. [CrossRef]
44. Zhang, C.; Chen, B.; Jiao, A.; Li, F.; Sun, N.; Zhang, G.; Zhang, J. MiR-663a inhibits tumor growth and invasion by regulating TGF-β1 in hepatocellular carcinoma. *BMC Cancer* **2018**, *18*, 1179. [CrossRef]

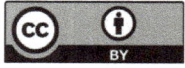

© 2020 by the authors. Licensee MDPI, Basel, Switzerland. This article is an open access article distributed under the terms and conditions of the Creative Commons Attribution (CC BY) license (http://creativecommons.org/licenses/by/4.0/).

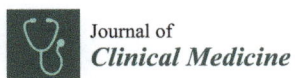

Article

Sex-Sparing Robot-Assisted Radical Cystectomy with Intracorporeal Padua Ileal Neobladder in Female: Surgical Technique, Perioperative, Oncologic and Functional Outcomes

Gabriele Tuderti [1,*], Riccardo Mastroianni [1,2], Simone Flammia [2], Mariaconsiglia Ferriero [1], Costantino Leonardo [2], Umberto Anceschi [1], Aldo Brassetti [1], Salvatore Guaglianone [1], Michele Gallucci [2] and Giuseppe Simone [1]

1. "Regina Elena" National Cancer Institute, Department of Urology, 00100 Rome, Italy; riccardomastroianniroma@gmail.com (R.M.); marilia.ferriero@gmail.com (M.F.); umberto.anceschi@gmail.com (U.A.); aldo.brassetti@gmail.com (A.B.); salvatore.guaglianone@ifo.gov.it (S.G.); puldet@gmail.com (G.S.)
2. "Sapienza" University of Rome, Department of Urology, 00100 Rome, Italy; roccosimone92@gmail.com (S.F.); costantino.leonardo@uniroma1.it (C.L.); michele.gallucci@ifo.gov.it (M.G.)
* Correspondence: gabriele.tuderti@gmail.com; Tel.: +39-3208234990

Received: 8 January 2020; Accepted: 14 February 2020; Published: 20 February 2020

Abstract: Our aim was to illustrate our technique of sex-sparing (SS)-robot-assisted radical cystectomy (RARC) in female patients receiving an intracorporeal neobladder (iN). From January 2013 to June 2018, 11 female patients underwent SS-RARC-iN at a single tertiary referral center. Inclusion criteria were a cT ≤ 2 N0 M0 bladder tumor at baseline imaging (CT or MRI) and an absence of tumors in the bladder neck, trigone and urethra at TURB. Baseline, perioperative, and outcomes at one year were reported. The median operative time was 255 min and the median hospital stay was seven days. Low-grade Clavien complications occurred in four patients (36.3%), while high-grade complications were not observed in any. Seven patients (63.7%) had an organ-confined disease at the pathologic specimen; nodal involvement and positive surgical margins were not detected in any of the cases. At a median follow-up of 28 months (IQR 14–51), no patients developed new onset of chronic kidney disease stage 3b. After one year, daytime and nighttime continence rates were 90.9% and 86.4% respectively. Quality of life as well as physical and emotional functioning improved significantly over time (all $p \leq 0.04$), while urinary symptoms and sexual function worsened at three months with a significant recovery taking place at one year (all $p \leq 0.04$). Overall, 8 out of 11 patients (72.7%) were sexually active at the 12-month evaluation. In select female patients, SS-RARC-iN is an oncologically sound procedure associated with favorable perioperative and functional outcomes.

Keywords: bladder cancer; female; intracorporeal neobladder; outcomes; radical cystectomy; robotic; sex-sparing

1. Introduction

Radical cystectomy (RC) with urinary diversion is the standard treatment for patients with muscle-invasive (MI) and high-risk non-muscle-invasive (NMI) urothelial carcinoma of the bladder and can offer an orthotopic neobladder (ON) diversion if technically and oncologically feasible [1].

Although bladder cancer (BCa) is more frequent among men, it remains the 17th most common cancer in women worldwide, with approximately 74,000 new diagnosed cases each year [2]. Moreover, women present an advanced stage at diagnosis more often, increasing the requirement of RC [3].

In female patients, the standard surgical procedure is represented by anterior pelvic exenteration including the removal of the bladder, ovaries, uterus, and anterior vaginal wall [1].

In this setting, when an ON is performed, the procedure can be associated with a considerable rate of voiding symptoms [4,5]. In addition, sexual dysfunction derived from such a highly demolitive surgical procedure is a key concern, especially in younger patients due to a significant impact on health-related quality of life (HRQoL) [6].

The improvement of imaging modalities, an increased knowledge of pelvic structure anatomy and function, and an advancement of surgical techniques have enabled less-destructive methods for treating high-risk BCa.

In this scenario, various types of pelvic-organ-preserving techniques, usually named "sex-sparing", have been proposed [5], aiming at the preservation of neurovascular bundles, vagina, and uterus, combining these techniques in order to optimize sexual and functional results without compromising oncological outcomes.

Functional outcomes of sex-sparing (sex) RC are essentially based on surgical dissection planes, with the sex-sparing approach being associated with the preservation of utero-vaginal hypogastric plexus, while during standard RC only rectal hypogastric plexus is preserved [7].

The Bern group were the first to describe the feasibility of nerve-sparing RC and ON replacement in female patients, highlighting the potential advantages which derive from preserving pelvic reproductive organs and their nervous structures both in terms of continence and urinary retention [7].

However, a recent systematic review aiming at the evaluation of the advantages and disadvantages of sexual-function-preserving RC and ON in female patients underlined the need for further and more robust comparisons between sex and standard RC as existing data are still immature [5].

Notwithstanding, for well-selected patients, sparing female reproductive organs during RC can be an oncologically safe procedure and can provide improved functional outcomes.

Accordingly, despite the widespread use of robot-assisted radical cystectomy (RARC), there is a paucity of data concerning outcomes of sex-RARC with intracorporeal ON (iON) performed in female patients.

In this paper we describe surgical steps of sex-RARC in female patients, highlighting differences with the standard technique and anatomical details of preservation of the inferior hypogastric plexus (IHP) and we report perioperative, pathologic, and functional outcomes.

2. Experimental Section

2.1. Patients

Our single-center Institutional-Review-Board-approved BCa database was queried for "Female", "RARC", "iON", and "Sex-sparing". Overall, 11 patients were treated between January 2013 and June 2018, with a minimum one year of follow-up. Inclusion criteria were a cT ≤ 2 N0 M0 bladder tumor at baseline imaging (CT or MRI) and an absence of tumors in the bladder neck, trigone, and urethra at transurethral resection of the bladder tumor (TURB). Exclusion criteria included any contraindication to ON. All subjects gave their written informed consent for inclusion before they participated in the study.

2.2. Surgical Technique

2.2.1. Sex-Sparing Robot-Assisted Radical Cystectomy

The patient was placed in a steep Trendelenburg position, and a six trocars access was performed as previously described [8].

Sex-RARC was performed replicating the principles of open technique described by Bhatta Dhar et al. [7]. After an incision of the posterior peritoneum up to the round ligament, the ureters were identified and meticulously isolated with a "no-touch" technique. The umbilical artery, uterine artery, superior and inferior vesical arteries, and vaginal branches were carefully prepared bilaterally.

Because the uterus was going to be spared, the peritoneum was incised at the level of the utero-vesical junction in order to deflect the uterus and develop a vesico-vaginal plane between the bladder and the anterior wall of the uterus. The vaginal wall dissection at the cervical level was performed in the anterior plane of the vagina at the 2 and 10 o'clock position in order to preserve the utero-vaginal and pararectal components of the IHP (highlighted in red and green colors respectively, in the video), while in the standard technique the dissection is usually performed dorsolaterally at the 4 and 8 o'clock position, preserving only the pararectal plexus and removing en bloc with the specimen and the utero-vaginal components of the IHP. The superior and inferior vesical arteries and veins were secured with Hem-o-lok clips (Teleflex, Wayne, PA, USA) and transected with LigaSure at their origin from the internal iliac vessels, while the uterine arteries and the vaginal branches directed to the paravaginal tissue were preserved. Both ureters were divided between Weck clips, and margins were sent for frozen sections. Next, the Retzius space was approached. Endopelvic fascia was incised very close to the bladder neck in order to reduce the risk of an accidental injury of neurovascular paraurethral structures, which is crucial for both sexual and continence functionality. The urethra was prepared and a sample was sent for frozen section. Bladder was secured in an endobag and extracted through a 3-cm prepubic incision.

2.2.2. Pelvic Lymph Node Dissection and Intracorporeal Orthotopic Neobladder

A meticulous separate package extending pelvic lymph node dissection (PLND) was performed, including obturator, internal, external, and common iliac nodes. Considering that superior hypogastric plexus (SHP) is usually located just below the aortic bifurcation, ventrally to the sacral promontory, presacral nodes are not removed. Moreover, lymphatic tissue medial to internal iliac arteries which is in close contact with uterine and vaginal vessels and with uterine and vaginal plexus is usually spared.

After RC and PLND, intracorporeal Padua ileal neobladder was performed as previously described [8].

2.3. Outcomes Evaluated

Collected demographic parameters were age, body mass index (BMI), gender, and American Society of Anesthesiologists (ASA) score. Clinical variables were preoperative eGFR, preoperative hemoglobin (Hgb), and neoadjuvant chemotherapy rate. Surgical outcomes reported consisted of operative time, Hgb at discharge, hospital stay, and complications according to the Clavien–Dindo system [9]. Pathological findings including pT stage, pN stage, histology, lymph node count, and the positive surgical margin status were analyzed. Functional outcomes assessed were the last eGFR, neobladder stones rate, the uretero-ileal strictures rate, and the need for intermittent self-catheterization. Daytime and nighttime continence recovery probabilities were assessed over time. EORTC QLQ-C30 and EORTC QLQ-BLM30 questionnaires were adopted to assess HRQoL and urinary symptoms respectively. Every item measured ranged in a score from 0 to 100. A Female Sexual Function Index (FSFI) questionnaire was adopted for sexual function assessment [10]. Each of the six sexual domains range in score from 0 to 6, with a maximum global score of 36. Questionnaires were administered at baseline, and at 3 and 12 month follow-up.

As supplementary data, we reported preoperative perioperative, pathologic and functional characteristics comparisons of sex-RARC and standard RARC cohorts.

2.4. Statistical Analysis

Descriptive analyses were used. Frequencies and proportions were reported for categorical variables. Medians and interquartile ranges (IQRs) were reported for continuously coded variables.

The Kaplan–Meier method was performed to report daytime and nighttime continence recovery probabilities. Continence rates were computed at 3, 6, 12 and 18 months after surgery.

Differences between questionnaires' domains scores evaluated at the baseline 3-month, and 1-year follow-up were assessed with the Friedman test.

In the supplementary outcomes, comparison, continuous, and categorical variables were compared with a Student's *t*-test and a chi-square test respectively. The Kaplan–Meier method was performed to compare daytime continence recovery probabilities between sex-RARC and standard RARC cohorts. Continence rates were computed at 3, 6, 12, and 18 months after surgery and the log-rank test was applied to assess any statistically significant differences between the two groups.

All *p*-values < 0.05 were considered statistically significant. Statistical analysis was performed using SPSS v24 (IBM Corp., Armonk, NY, USA).

3. Results

Baseline and clinical features were reported in Table 1. Median operative time was 255 min (IQR 250–399). The median hospital stay was 7 days (7–12). Low-grade Clavien complications occurred in four patients (36.3%) while high grade complications were not observed. Seven patients (63.7%) had an organ-confined disease at the pathologic specimen; nodal involvement and positive surgical margins were not detected in any case (Table 2).

All patients had a minimum follow-up period of one year. At a median follow-up of 28 months (IQR 14–51), no patient developed a new onset of chronic kidney disease stage 3b. One patient reported a neobladder stone formation, and one patient developed a ureteroileal anastomotic stricture and required robotic reimplantation 18 months following surgery (Table 2).

One-year daytime and nighttime continence recovery probability were 90.9% and 86.4%, respectively (Figure 1a,b). Three patients performed self-catheterization twice a day (early morning and before night rest).

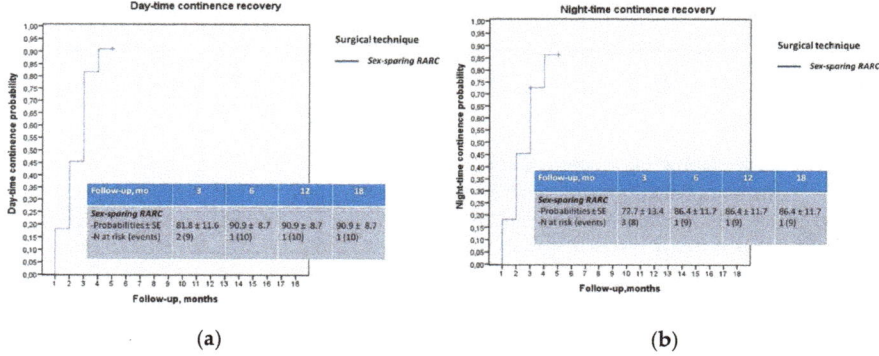

Figure 1. (a,b) Kaplan–Meier analysis reporting daytime and nighttime continence recovery probabilities.

Table 1. Baseline and clinical characteristics.

Patients, n 11	Sex-Sparing RARC
Age, year, mean (±SD)	47.1 (13)
BMI, mean (±SD)	23.1 (3.3)
ASA score, *n* (%)	
1	4 (36.4)
2	6 (54.6)
3	1 (9)
4	-
Preoperative eGFR, mL/min, mean (±SD)	84 (26.8)
Preoperative Hgb, g/dL, mean (±SD)	12.6 (1.9)
Neoadjuvant Chemotherapy, *n* (%)	4 (36.3)

Table 2. Perioperative, pathologic, oncologic and functional outcomes.

Patients	Sex-Sparing RARC (11)
Operative time, min, median (IQR)	255 (250–399)
Hgb at discharge, g/dL, median (IQR)	10.8 (9.1–11.9)
Hospital stay, days, median (IQR)	7 (7–12)
Complications, n (%)	4 (36.3)
Clavien Low grade (1–2)	4 (36.3)
Clavien High grade (≥3)	0 (0)
pT stage, n (%)	
0, a, is	6 (54.6)
1	1 (9.1)
2	-
3	4 (36.3)
4	-
pN stage, n (%)	
0	11 (100)
1	-
2	-
Lymph node count, mean (±SD)	26.2 (14.3)
Positive surgical margins, n (%)	0 (0)
Follow-up, months, median (IQR)	28 (14–51)
1-Year recurrence-free survival, n (%)	11 (100)
1-Year cancer-specific survival, n (%)	11 (100)
1-Year overall survival, n (%)	11 (100)
Last eGFR, mL/min, mean (±SD)	79.2 (23.7)
Ureteroileal strictures, pts (%)	1 (9)
Neobladder stones, n (%)	1 (9)
Need for intermittent self-catheterization, n (%)	3 (27.2)

Concerning the EORTC-QLQ-C30 questionnaire, global health status/quality of life, physical, and emotional functioning items improved significantly over time (all $p \leq 0.04$), while no differences were observed in any other items evaluated (all $p \geq 0.10$) (Supplementary Table S1, Figure 2).

According to the EORTC-QLQ-BLM30 questionnaire, specific for BCa, urinary symptoms worsened at three months with a significant recovery at one year ($p = 0.02$). Accordingly, when matching the baseline with 1-year scores, the values were comparable ($p = 0.08$) (Supplementary Table S2, Figure 2).

Finally, the FSFI global score and FSFI domains such as arousal, lubrication, orgasm, satisfaction, and pain worsened over the first three months with a subsequent improvement at one year (all $p \leq 0.04$). Moreover, comparing baseline vs. 1-year scores, arousal and orgasm domains experienced a complete recovery ($p = 0.10$ and $p = 0.10$, respectively), while lubrication, satisfaction, and pain domains, as well as FSFI global scores, experienced a satisfying improvement but were statistically significantly lower than baseline (all $p \leq 0.025$) (Supplementary Table S3, Figure 3). Overall, 8 out of 11 patients (72.7%) were sexually active at the 12-month evaluation.

As supplementary analysis, 36 standard RARC patients were compared with the sex-RARC cohort. The two cohorts were homogeneous for all baseline, clinical, and pathological features (all $p \geq 0.14$) except for age, with sex-sparing patients being significantly younger (47.1 vs. 61.7 years, $p < 0.001$) (Supplementary Tables S4 and S5).

Perioperative complications and hospital stay were comparable between groups ($p = 0.25$ and $p = 0.67$ respectively) (Supplementary Table S5).

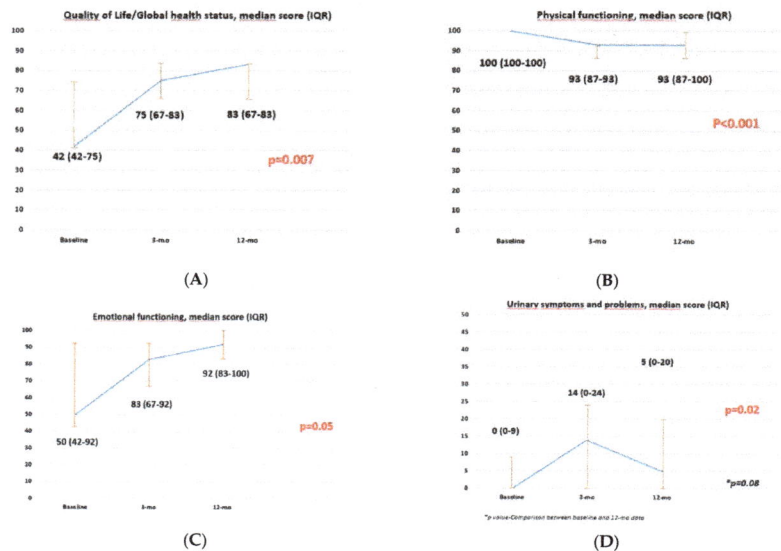

Figure 2. Graphs showing EORTC-QLQ-C30 and EORTC-QLQ-BLM30 questionnaire items displaying statistical significance according to the Friedman test. (**A**) Quality of Life/Global health status; (**B**) Emotional functioning; (**C**) Physical functioning; (**D**) Urinary symptoms and problems

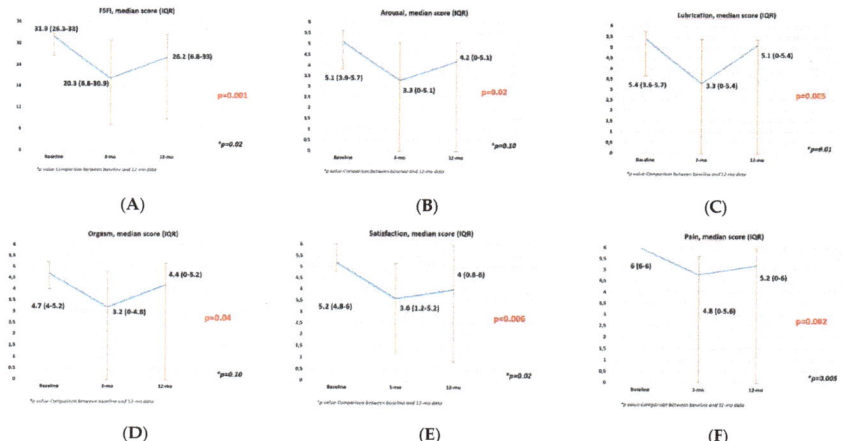

Figure 3. Graphs showing global Female Sexual Function Index (FSFI) and FSFI single domains questionnaire displaying statistical significance according to the Friedman test. (**A**) FSFI; (**B**) Arousal; (**C**) Lubrication; (**D**) Orgasm; (**E**) Satisfaction; (**F**) Pain.

With regard to functional outcomes, no significant differences were observed for the last estimated glomerular filtration rate ($p = 0.43$), neobladder stone formation rate ($p = 0.93$), and 1-year incidence of ureteroileal strictures ($p = 0.67$) (Supplementary Table S5). Daytime continence recovery probability was significantly higher in the sex-sparing cohort (1-year rate 90.9% vs. 74%, log-rank $p = 0.02$) (Supplementary Figure S1).

4. Discussion

Functional outcomes among women undergoing RC have been poorly addressed in the literature [11]. Urinary function is the most studied issue, although daytime and nighttime continence rates range significantly across studies due to a heterogeneity of definitions for continence, different inclusion criteria, and a lack of questionnaire adoption, as these are omitted in most studies [11]. In addition, Zahran et al. conducted a systematic review aiming to evaluate female sexual dysfunction post RC and urinary diversion, considering it an important predictor of HRQoL post RC. According to the 11 studies included, the most frequently detected sexual disorders were loss of sexual desire and orgasm disorders (49% and 39%, respectively) [12]. Notwithstanding, the authors called for the use of standardized tools in order to properly assess the outcomes of this technique from the patients' perspective and reported poor evidence from the available literature. Moreover, no data were available about RARC in females.

The concept of sex-RC in female patients was first introduced by the Bern team in 2007, when, in select female patients with an absence of invasive cancer at the level of the trigone or dorsolateral side walls of the bladder, they emphasized the functional advantages deriving from the preservation of the utero-vaginal hypogastric plexus, which is usually sacrificed in the standard procedure [7].

These results were corroborated by meticulous cadaveric studies elucidating topographic anatomic details of the nervous autonomic system in women, with their clinical nuances [13,14]. The SHP was identified as a single anatomical complex located below the aortic bifurcation, ventral to the sacral promontory. After the promontory, the SHP divides into right and left hypogastric nerves that more caudally plunge into the inferior pelvic IHP, composed by utero-vaginal, vesical, and rectal plexus.

As expected, preservation of these neural structures has an impact on recovery of urinary continence and on voiding function. Accordingly, data coming from gynecological studies report intrinsic sphincter deficiency resulting from hysterectomy as a consequence of urethral denervation after an extensive pelvic dissection [15,16]. Moreover, a pelvic autonomous nervous system affects all the domains of sexuality, such as sexual desire, arousal, lubrication, orgasm, satisfaction, and post-RC sexual dysfunction, often associated with pain disorders, such as dyspareunia, vulvodynia, and vaginismus, each being a consequence of autonomic and nociceptive nerve injuries, and a shortening or a narrowing of the vagina with an unavoidable negative impact on HRQoL [17].

In the literature, there are few existing series reporting sexual function results after sex-RC, all of them with an open approach and most of them with a small number of patients and without assessment of HRQoL through self-administered standardized questionnaires. Nandipati et al. focused on preservation of the lateral walls of the vagina, in which are embedded nervous fibers directed to the paraurethral tissue, involved in clitoral vascularization. In the small cohort of six women who underwent the sex-sparing approach, 12-month FSFI remained stable, while it declined in the standard RC group [18].

Furthermore, a significant improvement in all domains of the FSFI questionnaire has been reported in 13 sex-sparing RC patients evaluated at Mansoura Urology Department, with daytime and nighttime continence rates of 100% and 92%, respectively [19].

In this context, the EAU MIBCa Guideline Panel recently commissioned a systematic review aiming to assess the effect of sexual-function-preserving surgical techniques on outcomes in women receiving RC and ON substitution for BCa [5]. Sex-sparing approaches were found to be oncologically safe in well-selected patients, with sexual function appearing to be improved among those women undergoing gynecologic organ-preserving and nerve-sparing approaches. Nevertheless, most of the studies analyzed were retrospective and only contained a small number of patients [5]. Hence, according to EAU guidelines, data regarding sex RC in female patients are still considered immature and it is not yet considered a standard treatment, but an option to be taken into consideration for women highly motivated to preserve sexual function so long as strict oncologic inclusion criteria are met [1]. In addition, though the oncological equivalence of open and robotic RC has been extensively assessed, [20–22] and the robotic approach has been widely adopted in the male sex-sparing counterpart with excellent functional results [23], there are no reports on sex-RARC in female patients.

Hence, in this paper and in the accompanying video, we firstly described surgical steps of sex-RARC in female patients and reported perioperative and functional outcomes of our initial series with a minimum 1-year follow-up. In the video, we clearly highlight the differences with the standard technique with special attention paid to the preservation of the utero-vaginal component of the IHP. We strongly believe that robotic technology offers undebatable advantages in meticulously following and dissecting the appropriate surgical planes since IHP fibers are usually embedded in dense connective tissue, and consequently are not always easy to preserve. Despite the small cohort (11 patients), the excellent continence results (daytime 90.9% and nighttime 86.4% at one year) and the encouraging rate of sexually active patients (72.7% at one year) reflect the proper respect of the crucial anatomical structures and reinforce the efficacy of sex-RC in properly selected women. In addition, the oncological effectiveness with an absence of any recurrence corroborates our results.

Another important point of strength regarding the reliability of our results is our adoption of standardized questionnaires to assess the quality of life, urinary symptoms, and sexual activity (i.e., EORTC-C30, BLM30, and FSFI), which are rarely used in most studies. Moreover, the minimal invasiveness of the robotic approach represents a further issue to consider when considering young sexually and socially active women.

Furthermore, our technique may avoid devastating complications such as vaginal dehiscence and evisceration which have been reported after minimally invasive radical cystectomy [24,25].

Nevertheless, the present paper is not devoid of limitations. The small sample size, the strict inclusion criteria, and the need for advanced robotic surgical skills are significant limitations to a wide reproducibility of these outcomes in daily practice. Finally, BCa recurrence usually occurs within two years of radical cystectomy. In this respect, the follow-up duration might be inadequate.

5. Conclusions

In selected populations, sex-RARC-iN can be offered to female patients motivated to preserve sexual function as an oncologically safe procedure, associated with favorable functional outcomes. The meticulous anatomical preservation of utero-vaginal components of IHP represents the cornerstone of a quick and effective recovery of physiological functions in terms of urinary continence and sexual activity. A proper comparison of outcomes with the conventional RARC-iN technique requires properly designed prospective randomized trials.

Supplementary Materials: The following are available online at http://www.mdpi.com/2077-0383/9/2/577/s1. Table S1. Health-related quality of life assessment (EORTC QLQ-C30 questionnaire). Table S2. Bladder-cancer-specific quality of life EORTC QLQ-BLM30 questionnaire. Table S3. Female Sexual Function Index (FSFI) questionnaire. Table S4. Baseline and clinical characteristics of sex-sparing and standard RARC. Table S5. Perioperative, pathologic, and functional characteristics of sex-sparing and standard RARC. Figure S1. Kaplan–Meier analysis comparing day-time continence recovery probabilities between sex-sparing and standard RARC cohorts.

Author Contributions: Conceptualization, G.T, G.S.; methodology, G.T., R.M., G.S.; formal analysis, G.T.; data curation, R.M., S.F., M.F., C.L., U.A., A.B., S.G.; writing—original draft preparation, G.T., R.M.; writing—review and editing, G.T., G.S.; supervision, M.G., G.S. All authors have read and agreed to the published version of the manuscript.

Conflicts of Interest: The authors declare no conflicts of interest.

References

1. Witjes, J.A.; Lebret, T.; Compérat, E.; Cowan, N.C.; De Santis, M.; Bruins, H.M.; Hernández, V.; Espinos, E.L.; Dunn, J.; Rouanne, M.; et al. Updated 2016 EAU Guidelines on Muscle-invasive and Metastatic Bladder Cancer. *Eur. Urol.* **2017**, *71*, 462–475. [CrossRef]

2. Burger, M.; Catto, J.; Dalbagni, G.; Grossman, H.B.; Herr, H.; Karakiewicz, P.; Kassouf, W.; Kiemeney, L.; La Vecchia, C.; Shariat, S.; et al. Epidemiology and risk factors of urothelial bladder cancer. *Eur. Urol.* **2013**, *63*, 234–241. [CrossRef] [PubMed]
3. Mungan, N.; Aben, K.K.; Schoenberg, M.P.; Visser, O.; Coebergh, J.-W.W.; Witjes, J.; Kiemeney, L. Gender differences in stage-adjusted bladder cancer survival. *Urology* **2000**, *55*, 876–880. [CrossRef]
4. Granberg, C.F.; Boorjian, S.A.; Crispen, P.L.; Tollefson, M.K.; Farmer, S.A.; Frank, I.; Blute, M.L. Functional and oncological outcomes after orthotopic neobladder reconstruction in women. *BJU Int.* **2008**, *102*, 1551–1555. [CrossRef] [PubMed]
5. Veskimäe, E.; Neuzillet, Y.; Rouanne, M.; MacLennan, S.; Lam, T.B.L.; Yuan, Y.; Compérat, E.; Cowan, N.C.; Gakis, G.; Van Der Heijden, A.G.; et al. Systematic review of the oncological and functional outcomes of pelvic organ preserving radical cystectomy (RC) compared with standard RC in women who undergo curative surgery and orthotopic neobladder substitution for bladder cancer. *BJU Int.* **2017**, *120*, 12–24. [CrossRef]
6. Zippe, C.D.; Raina, R.; Shah, A.D.; Massanyi, E.Z.; Agarwal, A.; Ulchaker, J.; Jones, S.; Klein, E. Female sexual dysfunction after radical cystectomy: A new outcome measure. *Urology* **2004**, *63*, 1153–1157. [CrossRef]
7. Dhar, N.B.; Kessler, T.M.; Mills, R.D.; Burkhard, F.; Studer, U.E. Nerve-sparing radical cystectomy and orthotopic bladder replacement in female patients. *Eur. Urol.* **2007**, *52*, 1006–1014. [CrossRef]
8. Simone, G.; Papalia, R.; Misuraca, L.; Tuderti, G.; Minisola, F.; Ferriero, M.; Vallati, G.E.; Guaglianone, S.; Gallucci, M. Robotic Intracorporeal Padua Ileal Bladder: Surgical Technique, Perioperative, Oncologic and Functional Outcomes. *Eur. Urol.* **2018**, *73*, 934–940. [CrossRef]
9. Mitropoulos, D.; Artibani, W.; Biyani, C.S.; Jensen, J.B.; Rouprêt, M.; Truss, M. Validation of the Clavien-Dindo grading system in urology by the European Association of Urology Guidelines Ad Hoc Panel. *Eur. Urol. Focus* **2018**, *4*, 608–613. [CrossRef]
10. Rosen, R.; Brown, C.; Heiman, J.; Leiblum, S.; Meston, C.; Shabsigh, R.; Ferguson, D.; D'Agostino, R., Jr. The Female Sexual Function Index (FSFI): A multidimensional self-report instrument for the assessment of female sexual function. *J. Sex Marital. Ther.* **2000**, *26*, 191–208. [CrossRef]
11. Smith, A.B.; Crowell, K.; Woods, M.E.; Wallen, E.M.; Pruthi, R.S.; Nielsen, M.E.; Lee, C.T. Functional Outcomes Following Radical Cystectomy in Women with Bladder Cancer: A Systematic Review. *Eur. Urol. Focus* **2017**, *3*, 136–143. [CrossRef] [PubMed]
12. Zahran, M.H.; Fahmy, O.; El-Hefnawy, A.S.; Ali-El-Dein, B. Female sexual dysfunction post radical cystectomy and urinary diversion. *Climateric* **2016**, *19*, 546–550. [CrossRef] [PubMed]
13. Ripperda, C.M.; Jackson, L.A.; Phelan, J.N.; Carrick, K.S.; Corton, M.M. Anatomic relationships of the pelvic autonomic nervous system in female cadavers: Clinical applications to pelvic surgery. *Am. J. Obstet. Gynecol.* **2017**, *216*, 388.e1–388.e7. [CrossRef] [PubMed]
14. Mauroy, B.; Demondion, X.; Bizet, B.; Claret, A.; Mestdagh, P.; Hurt, C. The female inferior hypogastric (= pelvic) plexus: Anatomical and radiological description of the plexus and its afferences—Applications to pelvic surgery. *Surg. Radiol. Anat.* **2007**, *29*, 55–66. [CrossRef] [PubMed]
15. Mundy, A.R. An anatomical explanation for bladder dysfunction following rectal and uterine surgery. *Br. J. Urol.* **1982**, *54*, 501–504. [CrossRef] [PubMed]
16. Morgan, J.L.; O'Connell, H.E.; McGuire, E.J. Is intrinsicsphincter deficiency a complication of simple hysterectomy? *J. Urol.* **2000**, *164*, 767–769. [CrossRef]
17. Pederzoli, F.; Campbell, J.D.; Matsui, H.; Sopko, N.; Bivalacqua, T.J. Surgical Factors Associated with Male and Female Sexual Dysfunction After Radical Cystectomy: What Do We Know and How Can We Improve Outcomes? *Sex Med. Rev.* **2018**, *6*, 469–481. [CrossRef]
18. Nandipati, C.; Bhat, A.; Zippe, C.D. Neurovascualr preservation in female orthotopic radical cystectomy significantly improves sexual function. *Urology* **2006**, *67*, 185–186. [CrossRef]
19. Ali-El-Dein, B.; Mosbah, A.; Osman, Y.; El-Tabey, N.; Abdel-Latif, M.; Eraky, I.; Shaaban, A.A. Preservation of the internal genital organs during radical cystectomy in selected women with bladder cancer: A report on 15 cases with long term follow-up B. *Eur. J. Surg. Oncol.* **2013**, *39*, 358–364. [CrossRef]
20. Bochner, B.H.; Dalbagni, G.; Sjoberg, D.D.; Silberstein, J.; Keren Paz, G.E.; Donat, S.M.; Coleman, J.A.; Mathew, S.; Vickers, A.; Schnorr, G.C.; et al. Comparing open radical cystectomy and robot-assisted laparoscopic radical cystectomy: A randomized clinical trial. *Eur. Urol.* **2015**, *67*, 1042–1050. [CrossRef]

21. Moschini, M.; Soria, F.; Mathieu, R.; Xylinas, E.; D'Andrea, D.; Tan, W.S.; Kelly, J.D.; Simone, G.; Tuderti, G.; Meraney, A.; et al. Propensity-score-matched comparison of soft tissue surgical margins status between open and robotic-assisted radical cystectomy. *Urol. Oncol.* **2019**, *37*, 179.e1–179.e7. [CrossRef] [PubMed]
22. Simone, G.; Tuderti, G.; Misuraca, L.; Anceschi, U.; Ferriero, M.; Minisola, F.; Guaglianone, S.; Gallucci, M. Perioperative and mid-term oncologic outcomes of robotic assisted radical cystectomy with totally intracorporeal neobladder: Results of a propensity score matched comparison with open cohort from a single-centre series. *Eur. J. Surg. Oncol.* **2018**, *44*, 1432–1438. [CrossRef] [PubMed]
23. Asimakopoulos, A.D.; Campagna, A.; Gakis, G.; Montes, V.E.C.; Piechaud, T.; Hoepffner, J.-L.; Mugnier, C.; Gaston, R.; Corona, M.V.E. Nerve sparing robot-assisted radical cystectomy with intracorporeal bladder substitution in the male. *J. Urol.* **2016**, *196*, 1549–1557. [CrossRef] [PubMed]
24. Lin, F.C.; Medendorp, A.; Van Kuiken, M.; Mills, S.A.; Tarnay, C.M. Vaginal Dehiscence and Evisceration after Robotic-Assisted Radical Cystectomy: A Case Series and Review of the Literature. *Urology* **2019**, *134*, 90–96. [CrossRef]
25. Kanno, T.; Ito, K.; Sawada, A.; Saito, R.; Kobayashi, T.; Yamada, H.; Inoue, T.; Ogawa, O. Complications and reoperations after laparoscopic radical cystectomy in a Japanese multicenter cohort. *Int. J. Urol.* **2019**, *26*, 493–498. [CrossRef]

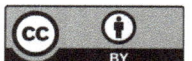

© 2020 by the authors. Licensee MDPI, Basel, Switzerland. This article is an open access article distributed under the terms and conditions of the Creative Commons Attribution (CC BY) license (http://creativecommons.org/licenses/by/4.0/).

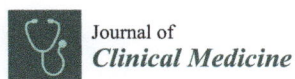

Article

Clear Cell Adenocarcinoma of the Urinary Bladder Is a Glycogen-Rich Tumor with Poorer Prognosis

Zhengqiu Zhou [1], Connor J. Kinslow [2], Peng Wang [3], Bin Huang [4], Simon K. Cheng [2,5], Israel Deutsch [2,5], Matthew S. Gentry [1,6] and Ramon C. Sun [6,7,*]

[1] Department of Molecular and Cellular Biochemistry, University of Kentucky College of Medicine, Lexington, KY 40536, USA; zhengqiu.zhou@uky.edu (Z.Z.); matthew.gentry@uky.edu (M.S.G.)
[2] Department of Radiation Oncology, Vagelos College of Physicians and Surgeons, Columbia University Irving Medical Center, New York, NY 10032, USA; cjk2151@cumc.columbia.edu (C.J.K.); sc3225@cumc.columbia.edu (S.K.C.); id2182@cumc.columbia.edu (I.D.)
[3] Division of Medical Oncology, Department of Internal Medicine, College of Medicine, University of Kentucky, Lexington, KY 40536, USA; p.wang@uky.edu
[4] Department of Biostatistics, College of Public Health, University of Kentucky, Lexington, KY 40536, USA; bhuang@kcr.uky.edu
[5] Herbert Irving Comprehensive Cancer Center, Vagelos College of Physicians and Surgeons, Columbia University Irving Medical Center, New York, NY 10032, USA
[6] Markey Cancer Center, University of Kentucky, Lexington, KY 40536, USA
[7] Department of Neuroscience, University of Kentucky College of Medicine, Lexington, KY 40536, USA
* Correspondence: ramon.sun@uky.edu

Received: 3 December 2019; Accepted: 30 December 2019; Published: 3 January 2020

Abstract: Clear cell adenocarcinoma (CCA) is a rare variant of urinary bladder carcinoma with a glycogen-rich phenotype and unknown prognosis. Using the National Cancer Institute's surveillance, epidemiology, and end results (SEER) program database, we documented recent trends in incidence, mortality, demographical characteristics, and survival on this rare subtype of urinary bladder cancer. The overall age-adjusted incidence and mortality of CCA was 0.087 (95% confidence interval (CI): 0.069–0.107) and 0.064 (95% CI: 0.049–0.081) respectively per million population. In comparison to non-CCAs, CCAs were more commonly associated with younger age (<60 years old, $p = 0.005$), female ($p < 0.001$), black ethnicity ($p = 0.001$), grade III ($p < 0.001$), and higher AJCC 6th staging ($p < 0.001$). In addition, CCA patients more frequently received complete cystectomy ($p < 0.001$) and beam radiation ($p < 0.001$) than non-CCA patients. Our study showed a poorer prognosis of CCAs compared to all other carcinomas of the urinary bladder ($p < 0.001$), accounted for by higher tumor staging of CCA cases. This study adds to the growing evidence that glycogen-rich cancers may have unique characteristics affecting tumor aggressiveness and patient prognosis. Additional mechanistic studies are needed to assess whether it's the excess glycogen that contributes to the higher stage at diagnosis.

Keywords: glycogen; clear-cell adenocarcinoma; urinary bladder; SEER program database

1. Introduction

Glycogen, a multibranched polymer of glucose, serves as our body's main form of carbohydrate storage [1]. In the past decade, glycogen has become well-established that, in addition to its role in maintaining metabolic homeostasis in normal cells, it also has a crucial role in promoting tumor growth, especially under adverse conditions [2]. Under hypoxic conditions, which are commonly encountered by tumors cells, expression of transcription factor HIF1α increases glycogen accumulation [3]. Cancer cells have been shown to mobilize this excess glycogen via a p38α mitogen-activated protein kinase pathway to fuel cellular proliferation and metastasis [4]. Glycogen has also been proposed to maintain the Warburg effect in tumor cells, providing a mechanism for survival during nutrient deprivation [5]. Furthermore, glycogen's inability to metabolize glycogen through small molecule inhibitors was able to induce apoptosis or senescence in tumor cells [6,7]. Altogether, cancer cells utilize glycogen as a way to alter its metabolic programing in order to adapt to the adverse tumor microenvironment and maintain tumor growth.

Aberrant glycogen deposits have been identified in tumors from multiple origins, including cancers of the breast, kidney, uterus, lung, head and neck, bladder, ovary, skin, brain and colorectal tumors [8–12]. They are often identified as "clear cell" due to the transparent and ovoid appearance seen on histological staining. A poorer prognosis has been documented in clear cell carcinomas of the kidney [13], uterus [14], ovaries [15] and breast [16]. However, due to the rarity of some these tumors, the prognostic implications in other types of "clear cell" cancers remain unclear.

Clear cell adenocarcinoma of the urinary bladder (CCA) is a rare histological growth pattern first reported by Dow and Young in 1968 [17]. These tumors contain sheets of uniform ovoid cells with clear cytoplasm containing abundant glycogen [18,19]. Since there are no distinguishing symptoms of CCA, diagnosis is based on histopathological identification of these characteristics. Due to its rarity, information on the characteristics and prognosis of CCA have been limited to case reports, with less than 50 cases reported to date [19–21]. The largest existing literature review was performed by Lu et al., consisting of 38 case reports [21]. The review supported surgical resection as initial treatment for CCA and noted a possible increase in metastasis risk compared to urothelial carcinomas. However, the study determined that the prognosis of CCA was unclear as longer follow up periods were needed to more accurately assess survival characteristics [21]. No incidence and mortality data have been reported yet.

As the first large-scale study to date, we utilized the National Cancer Institute's surveillance, epidemiology, and end results (SEER) program database to conduct a retrospective assessment of incidence, mortality, demographics, and survival for CCA. Based on the previous literature that has shown a link between glycogen rich tumors and tumor aggressiveness [13–16], our study aimed to assess whether similar prognostic outcomes exist for CCAs. Using 91 cases of CCA and 205,106 cases of other urinary bladder cancers (non-CCA) obtained from the SEER Program database, we identified a poorer prognosis attributed to higher staging at time for diagnosis for CCAs. Our study contributes to the growing body of evidence revealing a possible link between glycogen and tumor aggressiveness.

2. Experimental Section

2.1. Data Source

The SEER Program is the National Cancer Institute's authoritative source of information on cancer incidence and survival capturing approximately 34.6% of the US population [22]. It is populated with high quality population-based data from national cancer registries. Vital status is updated annually and routinely undergoes quality-control checks.

2.2. Sample Selection and Coding

Age-adjusted incidence and mortality rates were calculated using the SEER*Stat Software (Version 8.3.6, National Cancer Institute, Bethesda, MD, USA) using all 91 cases of malignant cases of CCA of the urinary bladder and 205, 106 cases of non-CCA from 2004 to 2015 from the SEER Program database [23,24]. Incidence and mortality were age-adjusted by standardizing to the 2000 United States Census population. All other data collection and analysis were conducted as described previously [16,25]. We obtained the November, 2015 submission [26] and November, 2017 submission [27] from the SEER Program database and merged all identified cases of malignant cancers of the bladder identified by International Classification of Diseases-O-3 (ICD-O-3) codes C67.0–C67.9 from January 2004 to December 2015. Carcinomas of the bladder were determined based on the adapted classification scheme for adolescents and young adults. Cases of clear cell adenocarcinoma were identified by ICD-O-3 code 8310.

The following variables were collected and coded: AYA site recode, primary site, ICD-O-3 histology, age at diagnosis, sex, race, grade, American Joint Commission on Cancer (AJCC) 6th Edition Staging, AJCC 6th Edition TNM system, survival months, vital status, bone metastasis at diagnosis, brain metastasis at diagnosis, liver metastasis at diagnosis, lung metastasis at diagnosis, surgery, and radiation. Cases of AJCC 6th stage 0a and 0is were merged and referred to as "stage 0". Ta, Tis were merged and referred to as "Ta/Tis". T1, T1a, T1b, T1 NOS were merged and collectively referred to as "T1". T2, T2a, T2b, T2 NOS were merged and collectively referred to as "T2". T3, T3a, T3b, T3c, T3 NOS were merged and collectively referred to as "T3". T4, T4a, T4b, T4 NOS were merged and collectively referred to as "T4". The surgery codes 10 (local tumor destruction), 20 (local tumor excision), and 30 (partial cystectomy) were merged and collectively referred to as "local procedure/partial cystectomy". Surgical codes 50 (simple/total/complete cystectomy), 60 (complete cystectomy with reconstruction), and 70 (pelvic exenteration) were combined, and collectively referred to as "complete cystectomy". Surgical codes 80 (cystectomy, NOS) and 90 (surgery, NOS) were combined and collectively referred to as "surgery, NOS". Detailed SEER database surgery codes are available at (https://seer.cancer.gov/manuals/2018/appendixc.html). Cases diagnosed at autopsy or that could have 0 days of follow-up were excluded all analyses except for incidence and mortality calculations.

2.3. Statistical Analysis

All statistical analysis was carried out using the IBM SPSS Statistics software package (version 25, International Business Machines Corporation, Armonk, NY, USA). The significance of incidence and mortality trends were calculated using linear regression analysis. Differences in demographic and clinical characteristics between CCA and non-CCA were determined using the Pearson's chi-square test. Median survival times were determined using the Kaplan–Meier method, and the significance was determined using the log-rank test. Multivariable analyses of overall survival were conducted using the Cox proportional hazards ratios (HR) model. Corresponding HR and 95% confidence intervals (CI) were estimated from the model. Two-tailed p-values < 0.05 were considered statistically significant.

3. Results

3.1. Incidence and Mortality of CCA

To assess recent trends in the incidence and mortality of CCA, we queried all cases of CCA from 2004 to 2015 in the SEER Program database. Over this period, the age-adjusted the incidence of CCA was 0.087 individuals per 1,000,000 (Supplementary Table S1). Our analysis suggested a downward trend in incidence over this period—a shift from 0.062 per 1,000,000 in 2004 to 0.057 per 1,000,000 individuals in 2015 with an annual decrease rate of 0.003. However, this trend was non-significant (p = 0.178, Supplementary Figure S1A). We further assessed incidence separated by gender (Supplementary Table S1). The incidence of CCA among female and males were similar, with a slight female predominance—0.091 and 0.084 per 10,000,000 for females and males respectively from 2004 to 2015 (Supplementary Table S1).

The mortality rate from 2004–2015 was 0.064 individuals per 1,000,000 with an increasing trend of 0.002 per year. This trend was also non-significant (p = 0.477, Supplementary Figure S1B, Supplementary Table S1). When separated by gender, male with CCA had higher mortality rate of 0.074 compared to 0.058 in females per 1,000,000 individuals (Table S1).

3.2. Demographics and Clinical Characteristics

To compare demographical and clinical characteristics of CCA to non-CCA cancers of the urinary bladder, we utilized cases of malignant carcinomas of the urinary bladder from 2004, when AJCC 6th staging information became available, to 2015, the most recent data available at time of analysis. We obtained 205,197 cases of malignant urinary bladder carcinoma. Of these, 91 cases (0.04%) were identified as CCA. The median follow-up time was 19 months with 45 deaths in these CCA patients.

Amongst 205,106 cases of non-CCA patients, the median follow-up time was 23 months, with 68,951 recorded deaths. The median age at diagnosis of CCA was 70 years old and median age at diagnosis was 72 years old in non-CCA patients.

The demographical and clinical characteristics of the patient population are summarized in Table 1. Our results showed that CCA patients were more likely to be younger age (<60 years of age; $p = 0.005$), female ($p < 0.001$) and black ($p = 0.001$) than non-CCA patients. The larger proportion of female patients is consistent with our incidence analysis. CCA patients also had higher grade ($p < 0.001$), higher AJCC 6th staging ($p < 0.001$) including TNM staging (p values for T, N, M stage were $p < 0.001$, $p < 0.001$ and $p < 0.001$, respectively). The primary site of tumor location was significantly different between CCA and non-CCA patients ($p < 0.001$); CCA patients were more likely to have tumors in the trigone of bladder, bladder neck and urachus, whereas non-CCA tumors appeared mostly in the lateral wall of bladder. As expected with more advanced tumor staging, CCA patients showed higher likelihood of brain ($p < 0.001$) and liver ($p = 0.028$) metastasis. However, very few cases with metastasis were available; only a single case was available for brain metastasis and two cases for liver metastasis. Furthermore, our data showed that non-CCA patients were more likely to receive fewer radical treatments such as local procedure or partial cystectomy, while more CCA patients received complete cystectomies ($p < 0.001$). The majority of non-CCA patients did not receive radiation, while a greater number of CCA patients received beam radiation ($p < 0.001$).

Table 1. Demographical and clinical characteristics comparing clear cell adenocarcinoma to other carcinomas of the urinary bladder.

		Clear Cell Adenocarcinoma ($N = 91$)		Non-Clear Cell Adenocarcinoma ($N = 205,106$)		
		Count	%	Count	%	p-Value
Age	0–60	27	29.7	37,649	18.4	0.005
	61+	64	70.3	167,457	81.6	
Sex	Female	54	59.3	49,241	24.0	<0.001
	Male	37	40.7	155,865	76.0	
Race	White	77	84.6	182,492	89.0	0.001
	Black	13	14.3	11,519	5.6	
	Other	1	1.1	8588	4.2	
	Unknown	0	0.0	2507	1.2	
Tumor primary site	Trigone of bladder	9	9.9	12,765	6.2	<0.001
	Dome of bladder	4	4.4	7213	3.5	
	Lateral wall of bladder	6	6.6	41,041	20.0	
	Anterior wall of bladder	5	5.5	4334	2.1	
	Posterior wall of bladder	7	7.7	18,819	9.2	
	Bladder neck	10	11.0	6354	3.1	
	Ureteric orifice	4	4.4	7820	3.8	
	Urachus	1	1.1	310	0.2	
	Overlapping lesion of bladder	13	14.3	21,112	10.3	
	Bladder, NOS	32	35.2	85,338	41.6	
Grade	Grade I	0	0.0	23,684	11.5	<0.001
	Grade II	5	5.5	48,123	23.5	
	Grade III	22	24.2	35,849	17.5	
	Grade IV	25	27.5	59,477	29.0	
	Unknown	39	42.9	37,973	18.5	

Table 1. Cont.

		Clear Cell Adenocarcinoma (N = 91)		Non-Clear Cell Adenocarcinoma (N = 205,106)		
		Count	%	Count	%	p-Value
AJCC 6th stage	Stage 0	2	2.2	105,545	51.5	<0.001
	Stage 1	22	24.2	46,332	22.6	
	Stage 2	28	30.8	23,463	11.4	
	Stage 3	9	9.9	8157	4.0	
	Stage 4	17	18.7	14,012	6.8	
	Unknown	13	14.3	7597	3.7	
T stage	Tis/Ta	2	2.2	105,545	51.5	<0.001
	T0	0	0.0	91	0.0	
	T1	26	28.6	49,221	24.0	
	T2	35	38.5	28,776	14.0	
	T3	7	7.7	8046	3.9	
	T4	11	12.1	7713	3.8	
	Unknown	10	11.0	5714	2.8	
N stage	N0	70	76.9	189,973	92.6	<0.001
	N1	2	2.2	3994	1.9	
	N2	6	6.6	3806	1.9	
	N3	1	1.1	166	0.1	
	Unknown	12	13.2	7167	3.5	
M stage	M0	75	82.4	193,071	94.1	<0.001
	M1	11	12.1	7565	3.7	
	Unknown	5	5.5	4470	2.2	
Bone metastasis [a]	No	42	97.7	102,083	97.0	0.697
	Yes	0	0.0	1432	1.4	
	Unknown	1	2.3	1698	1.6	
Brain metastasis [a]	No	41	95.3	103,393	98.3	<0.001
	Yes	1	2.3	122	0.1	
	Unknown	1	2.3	1698	1.6	
Liver metastasis [a]	No	40	93.0	102,600	97.5	0.028
	Yes	2	4.7	926	0.9	
	Unknown	1	2.3	1687	1.6	
Lung metastasis [a]	No	41	95.3	102,153	97.1	0.771
	Yes	1	2.3	1327	1.3	
	Unknown	1	2.3	1733	1.6	
Type of surgical procedure	No surgery	8	8.8	15,265	7.4	<0.001
	Local procedure/partial cystectomy	60	65.9	170,325	83.0	
	Complete cystectomy	22	24.2	18,327	8.9	
	Surgery NOS	0	0.0	504	0.2	
	Unknown if surgery performed	1	1.1	685	0.3	
Type of radiation [b]	None	67	85.9	160,440	94.6	<0.001
	Beam radiation	9	11.5	7485	4.4	
	Other radiation	1	1.3	219	0.1	
	Unknown if radiation received	1	1.3	1389	0.8	

Bolded are statistically significant p-values when comparing between clear cell adenocarcinoma to other carcinomas of the urinary bladder. NA—not applicable. [a] Variable only available for cases diagnosed after 2010. [b] Variable only available for cases diagnosed before 2013.

3.3. Survival

The median survival for CCA patients was 34 months with 5- and 10-year survival rates of 41%, 30%, respectively. The median survival for non-CCA patients was 87 months, with corresponding 5- and 10-year survival rates of 61% and 44%, respectively (Figure 1, $p < 0.001$). Using multivariable analysis accounting for age, sex, race, AJCC 6th stage, tumor grade, surgery, and radiation treatment, survival for CCA patients was no longer significantly poorer than non-CCA patients (HR: 0.93; 95% CI: 0.69–1.255; $p = 0.636$, Supplementary Table S2 left half). However, when staging was removed from same multivariable analysis, CCA survival remained significantly shorter than non-CCA patients (HR: 1.435, 95% CI: 1.064–1.936, $p = 0.018$, Supplementary Table S2 right half). Therefore, the histological subtype CCA is not an independent prognostic factor for survival, but instead, it is the more advanced staging in CCA patients accounts for the survival difference between CCA and non-CCA patients.

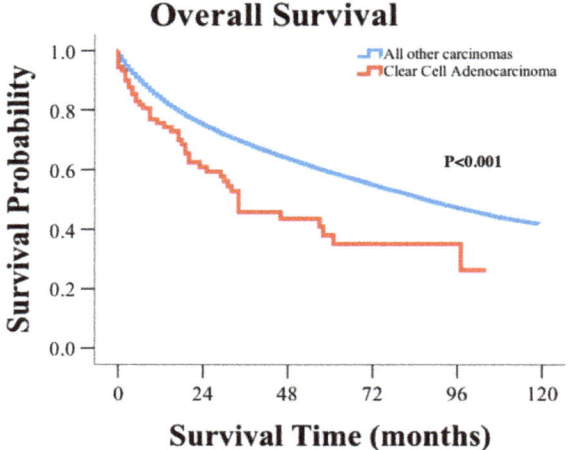

Number at Risk.

Survival months	0	24	48	72	96	120
CCA	205,106	100,972	63,338	35,862	15,121	0
Non-CCA	91	39	19	9	4	0

Figure 1. Kaplan–Meier curve and risk table of clear cell adenocarcinoma in comparison to other carcinomas of the urinary bladder.

To further confirm our finding that the worse prognosis is attributable for the higher staging, we stratified our CCA cases according to AJCC 6th staging and compared survival in patients with non-muscle invasive (AJCC 6th stage 0 and I), muscle-invasive (AJCC 6th stage II and III) and metastatic (AJCC 6th stage IV) pathology. As suspected, when stratified by non-muscle invasive, muscle-invasive, and metastatic cases, the survival durations were no longer significantly different between CCA and non-CCA cases (Table 2, $p = 0.654$, $p = 0.653$, $p = 0.091$ respectively).

Table 2. Survival comparison between clear cell adenocarcinoma and other urinary bladder cancers stratified by stage.

		Median Survival	95% Confidence Interval		p-Value
			Lower Bound	Upper Bound	
Non-muscle invasive (Stage 0–1)	Non-CCA	119			0.654
	CCA				
Muscle invasive (Stage 2–3)	Non-CCA	25	24.263	25.737	0.653
	CCA	32	16.308	47.692	
Metastatic (Stage 4)	Non-CCA	9	8.736	9.264	0.091
	CCA	18	13.315	22.685	

Moreover, when surgical procedure was assessed in each subgroup of patients stratified by staging, a significant difference in the survival of muscle-invasive CCA patients was observed. Patients receiving total cystectomy showed significantly greater survival probability than those receiving local procedures or partial cystectomy ($p = 0.028$, Figure 2A). However, for metastatic cases, no survival difference was observed based on surgical treatment received ($p = 0.269$, Figure 2B). Survival comparisons for non-muscle invasive cases were unable to be conducted due to the large number of censored events, i.e., patients that did not die during the follow-up period.

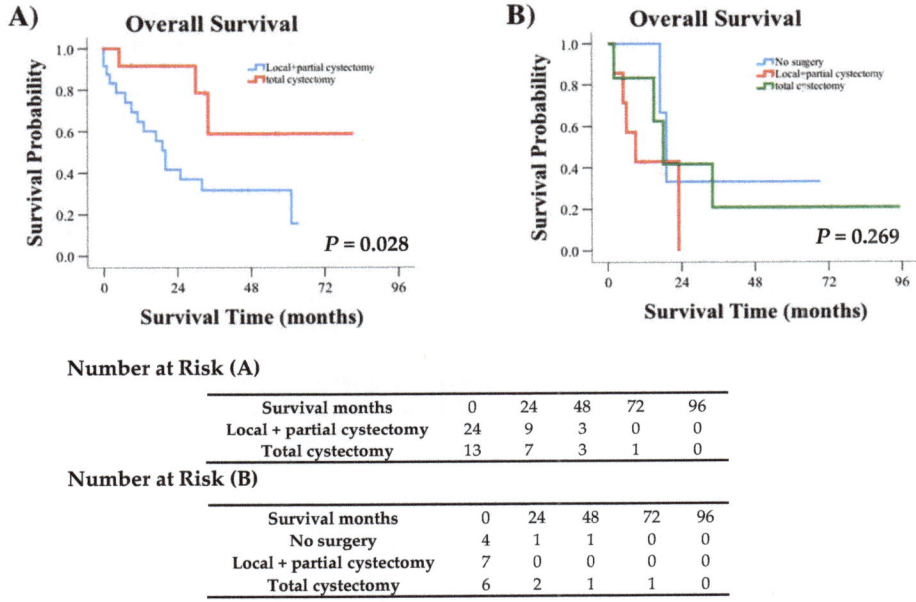

Figure 2. Kaplan–Meier curves and risk tables demonstrating survival for (**A**) muscle invasive cases of CCA defined by AJCC 6th stage II and III and (**B**) metastatic CCA cases defined by AJCC 6th stage IV.

4. Discussion

Using the SEER program database, we documented incidence, mortality, demographics, and survival on a rare subtype of urinary bladder cancer. We identified that CCAs were more commonly associated with younger age, higher grade, female gender, black ethnicity, and have a higher risk of brain and liver metastasis. Although it was not present in any of the cases reported in the SEER program database, bone metastasis in CCAs has been reported in several previously published case reports [28,29]. The most common location of CCA identified from our study was from trigone and bladder neck. This finding is consistent with previous reviews that also documented these as common tumor locations [21,28]. More importantly, our study showed a poorer prognosis of CCAs compared to all other carcinomas of the urinary bladder attributable to the higher tumor staging of the CCA cases. The poorer prognosis was irrespective of age, sex, race, grade, surgery and radiation treatment. In muscle invasive cases of CCA, type of surgical treatment was a significant factor in determining survival—There was improved survival when treated with complete cystectomies, which is consistent with standard of care for carcinomas of the urinary bladder [30].

The capability for glycogen to enhance tumor survival in adverse conditions may result in a faster invasion of CCA, hence, higher staging at diagnosis. Glycogen stores provide an excess glucose supply that can be utilized in the hypoxic conditions of tumor microenvironment [7]. The glycogen breakdown also generates nucleotides critical for cell proliferation such as NAPDH, an essential reducing agent, through the pentose phosphate pathway [7]. Furthermore, the glycogen shunt has been proposed to sustain the Warburg effect, a phenomenon that causes cells to use glucose in glycolysis instead of oxidative phosphorylation even in presence of plentiful oxygen in cells [31]. During periods of decreased glucose availability, the glycogen shunt sustains the production of glycolytic intermediates and ATP through the Warburg effect, hence maintaining tumor growth in nutrient deprived conditions [5].

Recently, the glycogen debranching enzyme amylo-α-1, 6-glucosidase, 4-α-glucanotransferase (AGL) was shown to have tumor suppressor functions in a model of urothelial bladder cancer [32]. Loss of AGL increased tumor growth in vitro and in xenografted tumors accompanied by an increase in abnormal glycogen structures (limit dextrin) and decrease in normal glycogen. The study also showed an increase in aerobic glycolysis and increased lactate, consistent with a shift towards the Warburg effect. Similar to our results, patients with reduced AGL expression was also associated with a decrease in overall survival, but was no longer predictive of survival when examined in a multivariate model that included age, sex, stage, and grade [32]. The similarities of our findings in CCA suggest that the manipulation of glycogen accumulations in urothelial bladder tumors may induce characteristics that mimic CCA.

While most urinary bladder cancers are male predominant [33], it was an interesting finding that CCA seemed to have a female predominance. The higher proportion of female patients supports a possible mullerian origin of CCA which has been previously proposed due to its association with endometriosis and histological resemblance to clear cell cancers of female genital tract [19,34]. Moreover, it is well known that females with urinary bladder cancers are generally diagnosed with more advanced disease and have poorer prognosis than males [33,35]. However, our findings suggested that it was CCA males instead who had higher mortality than females. Collectively, the gender disparity between CCA and other urinary bladder cancers suggest that CCA is an entity with differing characteristics to other urinary bladder cancers. More mechanistic and clinical studies are needed to improve our understanding of how gender and its associated factors relate to CCA pathology and prognosis.

At this time, no tailored therapy exists for CCA. Patients typically undergo some form of surgical resection such as transurethral resection, total cystectomy, partial cystectomy or radical surgery accompanied by chemotherapy and/or radiation [30]. Our study suggests that those with muscle invasive disease had survival benefit from total cystectomy rather than partial cystectomy, although prospective studies are needed to confirm these findings. Further understanding of cancer glycogen metabolism may help us with new avenues of tailored disease treatment. No information with regards to chemotherapy treatment was included in this manuscript due to a lack of reliable data in the SEER program database at this time.

5. Conclusions

As the first large-scale study to date, we assessed the incidence, mortality, demographical/clinical characteristics, and survival of CCA, a rare, glycogen-rich variant of urinary bladder cancer. We found a poorer prognosis of CCAs compared to all other carcinomas of the urinary bladder that was attributable to the higher staging of these tumors. However, the limitations of the study include the retrospective study design, small number of cases of interest (i.e., CCA) in comparison to control cases (i.e., non-CCA), and reliability of the SEER program database. Additional prospective clinical studies are needed to confirm these findings. Mechanistic studies that assess signaling pathways linking glycogen and rate of tumor growth would be beneficial for improving the understanding of the link between glycogen and poorer patient prognosis, and help to identify novel, targeted therapies for these glycogen-rich cancers.

Supplementary Materials: The following are available online at http://www.mdpi.com/2077-0383/9/1/138/s1, Table S1: Incidence and mortality of clear cell carcinoma of the urinary bladder from 2004–2015 per million population, Table S2: Multivariable analysis of survival for all urinary bladder patients, Figure S1: (**A**) Incidence of clear cell adenocarcinoma per million individuals in the US population. (**B**) Mortality of clear cell adenocarcinoma per million individuals in the US population.

Author Contributions: Z.Z. conducted the data analysis and drafted the manuscript. C.J.K. assisted with data analysis. P.W., S.K.C. and I.D. assisted in providing clinical insights for the manuscript. B.H. provided guidance on statistical analyses. M.S.G. and R.C.S. conceptualized the manuscript. All authors have read and agreed to the published version of the manuscript.

Funding: This study was supported by the St Baldrick's Career Development Award (Scholar), University of Kentucky Center for Cancer and Metabolism P20 GM121327, American Cancer Society institutional research grant #16-182-28, funding from the University of Kentucky Markey Cancer Center P30CA177558. Z.Z. is supported by the NIH National Center for Advancing Translational Sciences (grant number: UL1TR001998).

Acknowledgments: Special thanks to Gentry lab and Vander Kooi lab for the numerous discussions and continuous support.

Conflicts of Interest: The authors declare no conflict of interest. Cheng reports personal fees and non-financial support from AbbVie and Sanofi. Gentry and Sun report personal fees and non-financial support from Maze Therapeutics. However, AbbVie, Sanofi and Maze Therapeutics had no role in the design of the study; in the collection, analyses, or interpretation of data; in the writing of the manuscript, or in the decision to publish the results.

References and Notes

1. Young, L.E.A.; Brizzee, C.O.; Macedo, J.K.A.; Murphy, R.D.; Contreras, C.J.; DePaoli-Roach, A.A.; Roach, P.J.; Gentry, M.S.; Sun, R.C. Accurate and sensitive quantitation of glucose and glucose phosphates derived from storage carbohydrates by mass spectrometry. *Carbohydr. Polym.* **2019**, *230*, 115651. [CrossRef]
2. Schulze, A.; Harris, A.L. How cancer metabolism is tuned for proliferation and vulnerable to disruption. *Nature* **2012**, *491*, 364–373. [CrossRef] [PubMed]
3. Pelletier, J.; Bellot, G.; Gounon, P.; Lacas-Gervais, S.; Pouyssegur, J.; Mazure, N.M. Glycogen Synthesis is Induced in Hypoxia by the Hypoxia-Inducible Factor and Promotes Cancer Cell Survival. *Front. Oncol.* **2012**, *2*, 18. [CrossRef] [PubMed]
4. Curtis, M.; Kenny, H.A.; Ashcroft, B.; Mukherjee, A.; Johnson, A.; Zhang, Y.; Helou, Y.; Batlle, R.; Liu, X.; Gutierrez, N.; et al. Fibroblasts Mobilize Tumor Cell Glycogen to Promote Proliferation and Metastasis. *Cell Metab* **2019**, *29*, 141–155. [CrossRef] [PubMed]
5. Shulman, R.G.; Rothman, D.L. The Glycogen Shunt Maintains Glycolytic Homeostasis and the Warburg Effect in Cancer. *Trends Cancer* **2017**, *3*, 761–767. [CrossRef]
6. Lee, W.N.; Guo, P.; Lim, S.; Bassilian, S.; Lee, S.T.; Boren, J.; Cascante, M.; Go, V.L.; Boros, L.G. Metabolic sensitivity of pancreatic tumour cell apoptosis to glycogen phosphorylase inhibitor treatment. *Br. J. Cancer* **2004**, *91*, 2094–2100. [CrossRef] [PubMed]
7. Favaro, E.; Bensaad, K.; Chong, M.G.; Tennant, D.A.; Ferguson, D.J.; Snell, C.; Steers, G.; Turley, H.; Li, J.L.; Gunther, U.L.; et al. Glucose utilization via glycogen phosphorylase sustains proliferation and prevents premature senescence in cancer cells. *Cell Metab.* **2012**, *16*, 751–764. [CrossRef]
8. Rousset, M.; Zweibaum, A.; Fogh, J. Presence of Glycogen and Growth-related Variations in 58 Cultured Human Tumor Cell Lines of Various Tissue Origins. *Cancer Res.* **1981**, *41*, 1165–1170.
9. Rousset, M.; Chevalier, G.; Rousset, J.-P.; Dussaulx, E.; Zweibaum, A. Presence and Cell Growth-related Variations of Glycogen in Human Colorectal Adenocarcinoma Cell Lines in Culture. *Cancer Res.* **1979**, *39*, 531–534.
10. Staedel, C.; Beck, J.-P. Resurgence of glycogen synthesis and storage capacity in cultured hepatoma cells. *Cell Differ.* **1978**, *7*, 61–71. [CrossRef]
11. Altemus, M.A.; Yates, J.A.; Wu, Z.; Bao, L.; Merajver, S.D. Glycogen accumulation in aggressive breast cancers under hypoxia [abstract]. *Mol. Cell. Biol.* **2018**, *78* (Suppl. 13), 1446.
12. Sun, R.C.; Fan, T.W.M.; Deng, P.; Higashi, R.M.; Lane, A.N.; Le, A.-T.; Scott, T.L.; Sun, Q.; Warmoes, M.O.; Yang, Y. Noninvasive liquid diet delivery of stable isotopes into mouse models for deep metabolic network tracing. *Nat. Commun.* **2017**, *8*, 1646. [CrossRef] [PubMed]
13. Cheville, J.C.; Lohse, C.M.; Zincke, H.; Weaver, A.L.; Blute, M.L. Comparisons of outcome and prognostic features among histologic subtypes of renal cell carcinoma. *Am. J. Surg. Pathol.* **2003**, *27*, 612–624. [CrossRef] [PubMed]
14. Gadducci, A.; Cosio, S.; Spirito, N.; Cionini, L. Clear cell carcinoma of the endometrium: A biological and clinical enigma. *Anticancer Res.* **2010**, *30*, 1327–1334. [PubMed]
15. Sugiyama, T.; Kamura, T.; Kigawa, J.; Terakawa, N.; Kikuchi, Y.; Kita, T.; Suzuki, M.; Sato, I.; Taguchi, K. Clinical characteristics of clear cell carcinoma of the ovary: A distinct histologic type with poor prognosis and resistance to platinum-based chemotherapy. *Cancer* **2000**, *88*, 2584–2589. [CrossRef]

16. Zhou, Z.; Kinslow, C.J.; Hibshoosh, H.; Guo, H.; Cheng, S.K.; He, C.; Gentry, M.S.; Sun, R.C. Clinical Features, Survival and Prognostic Factors of Glycogen-Rich Clear Cell Carcinoma (GRCC) of the Breast in the U.S. Population. *J. Clin. Med.* **2019**, *8*, 246. [CrossRef]
17. Dow, J.A.; Young, J.D., Jr. Mesonephric adenocarcinoma of the bladder. *J. Urol.* **1968**, *100*, 466–469. [CrossRef]
18. Young, R.H.; Scully, R.E. Clear cell adenocarcinoma of the bladder and urethra. A report of three cases and review of the literature. *Am. J. Surg. Pathol.* **1985**, *9*, 816–826. [CrossRef]
19. Adeniran, A.J.; Tamboli, P. Clear cell adenocarcinoma of the urinary bladder: A short review. *Arch. Pathol. Lab. Med.* **2009**, *133*, 987–991.
20. Venyo, A.K. Primary Clear Cell Carcinoma of the Urinary Bladder. *Int. Sch. Res. Not.* **2014**, *2014*, 593826. [CrossRef]
21. Lu, J.; Xu, Z.; Jiang, F.; Wang, Y.; Hou, Y.; Wang, C.; Chen, Q. Primary clear cell adenocarcinoma of the bladder with recurrence: A case report and literature review. *World J. Surg. Oncol.* **2012**, *10*, 33. [CrossRef] [PubMed]
22. National Cancer Institute Surveillance. Epidemiology and End Result Program. Overview of the SEER Program. Available online: https://seer.cancer.gov/about/overview.html (accessed on 19 June 2016).
23. National Cancer Institute. DCCPS, Surveillance Research Program. Surveillance, Epidemiology, and End Results (SEER) Program (www.seer.cancer.gov). SEER*Stat Database: Incidence—SEER 18 Regs Research Data + Hurricane Katrina Impacted Louisiana Cases, Nov 2017 Sub (2000–2015) <Katrina/Rita Population Adjustment>—Linked To County Attributes—Total U.S., 1969–2016 Counties, released April 2018, based on the November 2017 Submission.
24. National Cancer Institute. DCCPS, Surveillance Research Program. Surveillance, Epidemiology, and End Results (SEER) Program (www.seer.cancer.gov) SEER*Stat Database: Incidence-Based Mortality—SEER 18 Regs (Excl Louisiana) Research Data, Nov 2017 Sub (2000–2015) <Katrina/Rita Population Adjustment>—Linked To County Attributes—Total U.S., 1969–2016 Counties, Released April 2018, based on the November 2017 Submission.
25. Kinslow, C.J.; Bruce, S.S.; Rae, A.I.; Sheth, S.A.; McKhann, G.M.; Sisti, M.B.; Bruce, J.N.; Sonabend, A.M.; Wang, T.J.C. Solitary-fibrous tumor/hemangiopericytoma of the central nervous system: A population-based study. *J. Neurooncol.* **2018**, *138*, 173–182. [CrossRef] [PubMed]
26. National Cancer Institute. DCCPS, Surveillance Research Program. Surveillance, Epidemiology, and End Results (SEER) Program (www.seer.cancer.gov) SEER*Stat Database: Incidence—SEER 18 Regs Research Data + Hurricane Katrina Impacted Louisiana Cases, Nov 2015 Sub (1973–2013 Varying)—Linked To County Attributes—Total U.S., 1969–2014 Counties, released April 2016, based on the November 2015 Submission.
27. National Cancer Institute. DCCPS, Surveillance Research Program. Surveillance, Epidemiology, and End Results (SEER) Program (www.seer.cancer.gov) SEER*Stat Database: Incidence—SEER 18 Regs Research Data + Hurricane Katrina Impacted Louisiana Cases, Nov 2017 Sub (1973–2015 Varying)—Linked To County Attributes—Total U.S., 1969–2016 Counties, released April 2018, based on the November 2017 Submission.
28. Matsuoka, Y.; Machida, T.; Oka, K.; Ishizaka, K. Clear cell adenocarcinoma of the urinary bladder inducing acute renal failure. *Int. J. Urol.* **2002**, *9*, 467–469. [CrossRef] [PubMed]
29. Honda, N.; Yamada, Y.; Nanaura, H.; Fukatsu, H.; Nonomura, H.; Hatano, Y. Mesonephric adenocarcinoma of the urinary bladder: A case report. *Hinyokika Kiyo* **2000**, *46*, 27–31. [PubMed]
30. National Comprehensive Cancer Network. NCCN Clinical Practice Guidelines in Oncology (NCCN Guidelines). Bladder Cancer. Version 1.2019. Available online: https://www.partnershipagainstcancer.ca/db-sage/sage20181257/# (accessed on 19 June 2018).
31. Warburg, O. On the origin of cancer cells. *Science* **1956**, *123*, 309–314. [CrossRef]
32. Guin, S.; Pollard, C.; Ru, Y.; Ritterson Lew, C.; Duex, J.E.; Dancik, G.; Owens, C.; Spencer, A.; Knight, S.; Holemon, H.; et al. Role in tumor growth of a glycogen debranching enzyme lost in glycogen storage disease. *J. Natl. Cancer Inst.* **2014**, *106*. [CrossRef]
33. Dobruch, J.; Daneshmand, S.; Fisch, M.; Lotan, Y.; Noon, A.P.; Resnick, M.J.; Shariat, S.F.; Zlotta, A.R.; Boorjian, S.A. Gender and Bladder Cancer: A Collaborative Review of Etiology, Biology, and Outcomes. *Eur. Urol.* **2016**, *69*, 300–310. [CrossRef]
34. Drew, P.A.; Murphy, W.M.; Civantos, F.; Speights, V.O. The histogenesis of clear cell adenocarcinoma of the lower urinary tract. Case series and review of the literature. *Hum. Pathol.* **1996**, *27*, 248–252. [CrossRef]

35. Cohn, J.A.; Vekhter, B.; Lyttle, C.; Steinberg, G.D.; Large, M.C. Sex disparities in diagnosis of bladder cancer after initial presentation with hematuria: A nationwide claims-based investigation. *Cancer* **2014**, *120*, 555–561. [CrossRef]

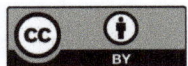 © 2020 by the authors. Licensee MDPI, Basel, Switzerland. This article is an open access article distributed under the terms and conditions of the Creative Commons Attribution (CC BY) license (http://creativecommons.org/licenses/by/4.0/).

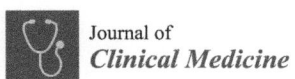

Article

Recovery from Anesthesia after Robotic-Assisted Radical Cystectomy: Two Different Reversals of Neuromuscular Blockade

Claudia Claroni [1,*], Marco Covotta [1], Giulia Torregiani [1], Maria Elena Marcelli [1], Gabriele Tuderti [2], Giuseppe Simone [2], Alessandro Scotto di Uccio [3], Antonio Zinilli [4] and Ester Forastiere [1]

1. Department of Anaesthesiology, IRCCS Regina Elena National Cancer Institute, 00144 Rome, Italy; marco.covotta@gmail.com (M.C.); giulia.torregiani@gmail.com (G.T.); mariaelena.marcelli@gmail.com (M.E.M.); ester.forastiere@ifo.gov.it (E.F.)
2. Department of Urology, IRCCS Regina Elena National Cancer Institute, 00144 Rome, Italy; gabriele.tuderti@gmail.com (G.T.); puldet@gmail.com (G.S.)
3. School of Medicine, University Hospital Center "Tor Vergata", 00133 Rome, Italy; allascotto@gmail.com
4. IRCrES, Research Institute on Sustainable Economic Growth of the National Research Council of Italy, 00185 Rome, Italy; antonio.zinilli@ircres.cnr.it
* Correspondence: claroni@icloud.com; Tel.: +39-3925786892; Fax: +39-0652662994

Received: 22 September 2019; Accepted: 21 October 2019; Published: 24 October 2019

Abstract: During robot-assisted radical cystectomy (RARC), specific surgical conditions (a steep Trendelenburg position, prolonged pneumoperitoneum, effective myoresolution until the final stages of surgery) can seriously impair the outcomes. The aim of the study was to evaluate the incidence of postoperative nausea and vomiting (PONV) and ileus and the quality of cognitive function at the awakening in two groups of patients undergoing different reversals. In this randomized trial, patients that were American Society of Anesthesiologists physical status (ASA) ≤III candidates for RARC for bladder cancer were randomized into two groups: In the sugammadex (S) group, patients received 2 mg/kg of sugammadex as reversal of neuromuscolar blockade; in the neostigmine (N) group, antagonization was obtained with neostigmine 0.04 mg/kg + atropine 0.02 mg/kg. PONV was evaluated at 30 min, 6 and 24 h after anesthesia. Postoperative cognitive functions and time to resumption of intestinal transit were also investigated. A total of 109 patients were analyzed (54 in the S group and 55 in the N group). The incidence of early PONV was lower in the S group but not statistically significant (S group 25.9% vs. N group 29%; $p = 0.711$). The Mini-Mental State test mean value was higher in the S group vs. the N group (1 h after surgery: 29.3 (29; 30) vs. 27.6 (27; 30), $p = 0.007$; 4 h after surgery: 29.5 (30; 30) vs. 28.4 (28; 30), $p = 0.05$). We did not observe a significant decrease of the PONV after sugammadex administration versus neostigmine use. The Mini-Mental State test mean value was greater in the S group.

Keywords: anesthesia recovery periods; bladder cancer; cognitive impairment; gamma-cyclodextrins; neuromuscular blockade; robotic radical cystectomy

1. Introduction

The diffusion of robot-assisted laparoscopic techniques has made it possible to perform surgical procedures with greater precision, and has reduced the need for transfusions, postoperative complications and hospitalization time [1]. In particular, robot-assisted radical cystectomy (RARC) has rapidly spread as the gold standard in the treatment of urothelial tumors, becoming a credible alternative to open cystectomy which is burdened by a high rate of complications [2].

Due to the particular surgical conditions and because of its recent application, there still are many anesthetic implications that must be examined thoroughly—patients have to satisfy specific clinical requirements, identified through careful anesthesiologic assessments [3].

During RARC, the anesthesiologist must be prepared to manage any hemodynamic, cerebrovascular and respiratory changes resulting from the surgical conditions that the robotic procedure requires, such as the prolonged use of pneumoperitoneum, the steep Trendelenburg position in which the patient is placed, and the lengthening of surgical times [4]. In addition, an effective myoresolution until the final stages of surgery is necessary to establish ideal surgical conditions [5] and the factors that can impair the quality and time of awakening [6]. To overcome this effect, a reversal of neuromuscular blockade (NMB) is routinely used in our clinical practice.

Currently, the effectiveness of the rocuronium/sugammadex combination for the reversal of the NMB has been widely demonstrated in terms of time and quality of neuromuscular and respiratory functions [7,8].

Neostigmine has been associated with an increased incidence of postoperative nausea and vomiting (PONV), although there is no definitive agreement on the need to avoid its use to reduce the incidence of PONV [9]. On the other hand, neostigmine has an important muscarinic effect on gastrointestinal (GI) receptors, and, by increasing the availability of acetylcholine, increases the GI motility.

In our study, we investigated if the use of a different kind of NMB reversal can influence the early postoperative period after a prolonged major surgery, such as RARC, affected by alterations on mechanical ventilation, cerebral perfusion, and vascular resistances [10]. Our aim is particularly focused on PONV and ileus, with attention to the recent collective effort to build an enhanced recovery after surgery (ERAS) path applicable specifically in the interventions of RARC [11].

The hypothesis is that the continuous infusion of rocuronium followed by sugammadex administration as NMB reversal in patients undergoing robotic radical cystectomy can improve the quality of awakening in terms of postoperative outcomes and cognitive function, compared to use of neostigmine as reversal.

The primary end point was to compare the incidence of PONV. Secondary end points were postoperative cognitive functions and time to resumption of intestinal transit (ROI).

2. Experimental Section

A mono-center prospective, two-arm parallel, randomized trial was conducted at the IRCCS Regina Elena National Cancer Institute. The study was approved by the Central Ethics Committee Lazio1, in May 2017, with Protocol n. CE/2288/17, and registered with ClinicalTrial.gov identifier NCT03144453. The clinical investigation was conducted according to the principles expressed in the Declaration of Helsinki.

2.1. Patients and Procedures

American Society of Anesthesiologists physical status (ASA) ≤III patients, candidates of RARC for bladder cancer, were enrolled after having given written informed consent. The exclusion criteria were age <18 years, inability to provide informed consent, BMI >30, and a history of cerebrovascular diseases.

Patients were randomly divided into two treatment groups by an operator who is not directly involved in the study using a specific dedicated software, developed in-house by a GW Basic (Microsoft Corporation, USA) programmer, which generates an assignment code verified immediately before arrival in the operating room. Surgeons were blinded to the intervention and blinded observers recorded the outcome.

In both groups, all patients were premedicated with midazolam 0.02 mg/kg and received dexamethasone 8 mg for anti-emesis. General anesthesia was induced with fentanyl 3–5 g/kg, propofol 2 mg/kg and a bolus of rocuronium 0.7 mg/kg was administered. After tracheal intubation, anesthesia was maintained with a mixture of sevoflurane/oxygen/air, adjusted to provide an end-tidal sevoflurane of 1.5–2 vol.%, remifentanil was adapted according to a target-controlled infusion (TCI) range of 2–4 ng/mL. Curarization started with rocuronium 5 g/kg/min and was set to maintain the post-tetanic count between 1 and 2. At the end of surgery, after skin closure, neuromuscular function was allowed to recover spontaneously and, at reappearance of the second twitch (T2), patients received a NMB reversal.

In the sugammadex group (S group), at T2 reappearance, patients received 2 mg/kg of sugammadex.

In the neostigmine group (N group), at T2 reappearance, antagonization was obtained with the standard NMB reversal agent: neostigmine 0.04 mg/kg and atropine 0.02 mg/kg to block the peripheral muscarinic side-effects of neostigmine.

All patients were extubated when the train-of-four (TOF) ratio was 0.9 or higher.

Nasogastric tube was removed after surgery, before the awakening.

In both groups, fluid therapy regimen was mainly restrictive, with a basal infusion of crystalloid variable from 2 to 4 mL/kg/h. Mean arterial blood pressure (MAP) was regulated by titrating remifentanil and fluid administration in order to maintain target values between 65 and 95 mmHg.

The standard monitoring for all patients consisted of continuous ECG, heart rate (HR) and MAP measurements, pulse oximetry (SpO2), inspired and expired gas, and capnometry. Neuromuscular function was measured using a TOF-Watch acceleromyograph (Organon ltd, Dublin, Ireland). After induction of general anesthesia, but before administering any NMB agent, the calibration of the acceleromyograph was performed according to the manufacturer's guidelines. The ulnar nerve received neuromuscular stimulation via two electrodes applied to the skin of the distal underarm, to the left and to the right of the ulnar nerve.

The surgical procedure was performed routinely following the standards of the Department of Urology at our hospital [12].

After surgery, patients requiring rescue anti-emetic therapy received ondansetron 4 mg, which was followed by metoclopramide 20 mg, if necessary.

All patients received intravenous morphine patient-controlled analgesia using the CADD®-Solis device (Smith Medical, Kent, UK) postoperatively. Patient-controlled analgesia was set on the demand mode without a loading dose. The dose of morphine was set at 0.02 mg/kg with a time-lock interval of 15 min.

All patients received morphine 0.07 mg/kg and 1000 mg acetaminophen at the time of surgical wound closure, followed by 1000 mg intravenous acetaminophen every 6 h for up to 5 days.

2.2. Measurements

Baseline data were collected, which included risk of PONV by Apfel score, neoadjuvant chemotherapy, and anxiety and depression by the Hospital Anxiety and Depression Scale.

During anesthesia, main parameters (MAP, HR, SpO2 and etCO2) and time to recovery from NMB reversal were recorded. Duration of surgery, amount of opioid consumption, comorbidities, and total amount of intensive care unit admission were also observed.

In the postoperative period, PONV (intended as number of episodes of nausea, vomiting or bloating) was evaluated after 30 min in post-anesthesia care unit (PACU), 6 and 24 h after anesthesia.

The assessment of consciousness at awakening and postoperative cognitive function was carried out by The Observer's Assessment of Alertness/Sedation Scale (OASS) at 15 min, 30 min, and 1 h after anesthesia, and through the Mini Mental State test (MMSt) at 1 and 4 h after anesthesia.

Early postoperative pulmonary failure (including bronchospasm, postoperative PaO2 <60 mmHg, a PaO2:FIO2 ratio ≥ 300 mmHg, or arterial oxyhemoglobin saturation measured with pulse oximetry <90% and requiring oxygen therapy) was noted after 24 h after anesthesia.

Time to resumption of intestinal transit, defined as time to return of peristalsis and time to first passage of flatus, antiemetics, and morphine consumption were recorded. Nurses detected peristalsis and gastrointestinal symptoms every 2 h and patients were asked to warn staff of the perception of bowel activity.

2.3. Statistical Analysis

The primary outcome was the cumulative incidence of PONV in the first 6 postoperative hours. Based on data from our department after this type of surgery using single-drug PONV prophylaxis and reversal of neuromuscular block with neostigmine, and according with previous study [13,14], we estimated that experience PONV would be 30% in neostigmine group and 8% in the sugammadex group. Based on power = 80% and a = 0.05, a sample size of 98 patients at least (n = 49 per group) was required.

For scores continuous, we used a two-sample Kolmogorov–Smirnov test, while for the ordinal categorical variable we used the Mann–Whitney U-test. P-values ≤ 0.05 were regarded as statistically significant. Data were analyzed using SPSS software (IBM, New York, United States).

3. Results

In the period between May 2017 and December 2018, a total of 109 patients were randomized: 54 patients to the S group and 55 to the N group.

The flowchart of the patients who participated in the study is demonstrated in Figure 1. The demographics and clinical characteristics were balanced for both treatment arms and are presented in Table 1. Intraoperative and perioperative data recorded are shown in Table 2.

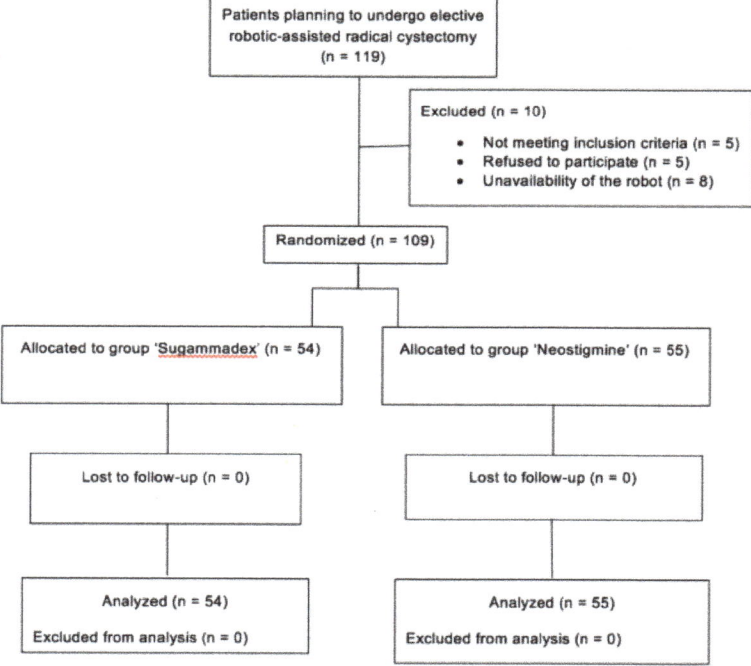

Figure 1. Patient disposition.

Time to recovery from TOF 2 to TOF ratio >0.9 was significantly lower in the S group. The incidence of early PONV was lower in the S group but not statistically significant (p = 0.711). The values were similar between the two groups for the incidence of late PONV.

The mean MMSt value was significantly higher in the S group compared with the N group at 1 h after anesthesia [mean and 25–75th percentile, 29.3 (29; 30) vs. 27.6 (27; 30); p = 0.007] and at 4 h after anesthesia [29.5 (30; 30) vs. 28.4 (28; 30); p = 0.048]. Thus, S group obtained better MMSt values during all measurements of time. The mean OASS value was significantly higher in the S group compared with the N group 1 h after the end of anesthesia (median and 25–75th percentile, 5 (5; 5) vs. 5 (4; 5); $p = 0.02$), but no differences were observed in the first measurement, 30 min after the end of anesthesia (Table 3).

Table 1. Demographic and clinical characteristics.

	S Group (n = 54)	N Group (n = 55)
Age (years), mean (SD)	62.8 (8.9)	60.2 (9.4)
BMI (kg/m^2), mean (SD)	26.3 (3.5)	26.2 (4)
Gender (n), male/female	42/12	40/14
ASA status (n): I/II/III	5/40/9	9/41/5
Apfel risk score (n): I/II/III/IV	20/30/4/0	19/32/4/0
Comorbidities, n (%)		
Hypertension	18 (33.3)	11 (20)
Dysthyroidism	3 (5.5)	4 (7.2)
Previous MI	5 (9.2)	2 (3.6)
Diabetes	6 (11.1)	3 (5.4)
COPD	3 (5.5)	2 (3.6)
Neoadiuvant chemotherapy, n (%)	14 (25.9)	11 (20)
Tumor stage (pT), n (%)		
Tis	8 (14.8)	7 (12.7)
Ta	3 (5.5)	3 (5.4)
T1	7 (13)	8 (14.8)
T2	13 (24)	14 (25.4)
T3	17 (31.4)	16 (29)
T4	6 (11.1)	7 (12.7)
HADS > 8, n (%)	25 (46.2)	27 (49)

BMI: body mass index; ASA: American Society of Anesthesiologists; COPD: chronic obstructive pulmonary disease; HADS: Hospital Anxiety and Depression Scale.

Table 2. Intraoperative and perioperative variables.

	S Group (n = 54)	N Group (n = 55)	p-Value
EtCO$_2$ (mmHg)	28.9 (3)	28.6 (3.4)	0.603
SpO$_2$ (%)	98.6 (1.3)	98.5 (1.5)	0.821
HR (bpm)	68.3 (15.1)	68.9 (13.9)	0.622
MAP (mmHg)	87 (15.3)	88.2 (15.5)	0.854
Estimated blood loss (mL)	209 (31)	218 (37)	0.200
Surgery time (min)	340.7 (80)	326.7 (81.9)	0.437
Anesthesia time (min)	378 (83)	361 (81)	0.526
Recovery time from TOF 2 to TOF Ratio > 0.9 (min)	3.2 (1)	8 (2.8)	<0.001 *
Early PONV 0–6 h, n (%)			
Cumulative incidence	14 (25.9)	16 (29)	0.711
Nausea	10 (18.5)	9 (16.3)	0.767
Vomiting	4 (7.4)	5 (9)	0.750
Late PONV 6–24 h, n (%)			
Cumulative incidence	10 (18.5)	11 (20)	0.845
Nausea	7 (13)	8 (14.5)	0.810
Vomiting	3 (5.5)	3 (5.4)	0.982
Antiemetics consumption (mg)			
Ondansetron	2.6 (3)	3.8 (4.4)	0.105
Metoclopramide	3.7 (4.9)	4.7 (5.7)	0.358
Morphine consumption (mg)			
0–6 h	3 (2.4)	3.7 (2.6)	0.154
0–24 h	6.2 (3)	5.5 (2.8)	0.177
Early postoperative pulmonary failure, n (%)	3 (5.5)	4 (7.2)	0.715
Time to resumption of intestinal transit, days (IQR)	3 (3–5)	3 (3–5)	0.761
Length of stay, days (IQR)	8 (7.5–12.25)	8 (6–12)	0.682

* p-value < 0.05; EtCO$_2$: end tidal CO$_2$; SpO$_2$: pulse oximetry; HR: heart rate; MAP: mean arterial pressure; TOF: train-of-four; PONV: postoperative nausea and vomiting; IQR: interquartile range.

Table 3. Consciousness at awakening and postoperative cognitive function.

	S Group (n = 54)	N Group (n = 55)	p-Value
	OASS ¢		
15 min	3 (3; 4)	3 (3; 4)	0.16
30 min	5 (4; 5)	4 (3; 5)	0.06
60 min	5 (5; 5)	5 (4; 5)	0.023 *
	MMSt #		
Preop	29.3 (30; 30)	29.2 (29; 30)	0.78
1 h	29.3 (29; 30)	27.6 (27; 30)	0.007 *
4 h	29.5 (30; 30)	28.4 (28; 30)	0.048 *

Data expressed as mean (IQR); ¢ Data expressed as median (IQR); p-value: two-sample Kolmogorov–Smirnov Test; * p-value < 0.05; OASS: Observer's Assessment of Alertness/Sedation Scale; MMSt: Mini Mental State test: IQR: interquartile range.

In Figure 2, we can observe that the trend in both MMSt and OASS is different between the two groups. The MMSt trend remained steadily higher since the awakening, while the values of OASS in S group were significantly increased after the first postoperative hour. The incidence of postoperative pulmonary failure was similar in each group. There were no significant differences between the groups for time to resumption of intestinal transit. Postoperative ondansetron and metoclopramide were similar in each group, as well as analgesic consumption.

Figure 2A. MMSt trend

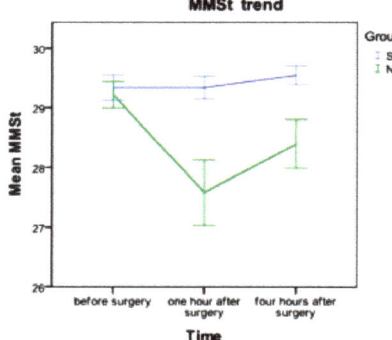
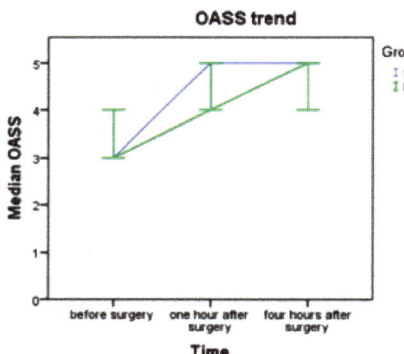

Figure 2B. OASS trend

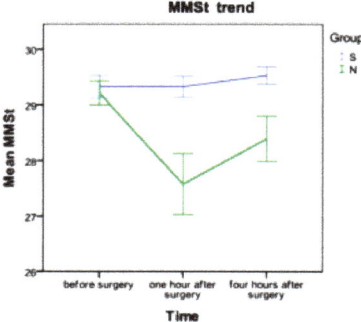
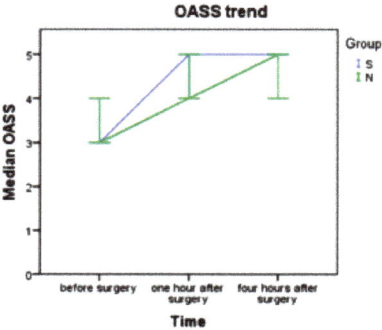

Figure 2. (A) MMSt and (B) OASS trend (error bars: 95% CI). Blue line: S group. Green line: N group.

4. Discussion

In our study, we attempted to evaluate the quality of recovery from anesthesia in two groups of patients who underwent robotic-assisted laparoscopic cystectomy. Prolonged myoresolution was carried out with continuous infusion of rocuronium: In one group, NMB reversal was obtained with sugammadex and in the other group, the association neostigmine/atropine was used.

Our results show that the incidence of PONV was greater in the N group, although non-statistically significant. Even time to resumption of intestinal transit was overlapping in the two groups.

In the past, studies concerning the reduction of PONV following the use of sugammadex have had conflicting results. Inhibiting cholinesterase action causes neostigmine increases concentration of acetylcholine, the principal excitatory neurotransmitter in the GI tract. Acetylcholine acts by increasing gastric secretions and esophageal pressure and increases the risk of symptoms such as nausea and vomiting, but also allows an increase in GI motility [15]. The prevention of PONV and the rapid restoration of intestinal function are fundamental topics in the development of ERAS protocols, which have shown efficacy in reducing complications and improving outcomes in many surgeries [16]. Nowadays, there are no definitive protocols specific to robotic surgery, and protocols applied in colorectal surgery are often used for cystectomy [10].

Our results agree with those of Peach et al. [17], which, in a large clinical trial of 304 women, did not find a lower incidence of PONV with the use of sugammadex compared with neostigmine. In contrast, Yağan et al. [13] found that the use of sugammadex had lower incidences of PONV in the first postoperative hour and less anti-emetic use at 24 h. In addition, in the study by Koyuncu et al. [18], sugammadex reduces PONV compared with neostigmine and atropine, but only slightly and transiently. While in the Yağan study [13], the population had undergone various types of surgery (more than half underwent head and neck surgery) and in the Koyuncu study [18] patient were candidates for extremity surgery, in the Peach study [17] patients underwent laparoscopic surgery, which, as in robotic cystectomy, involves a certain degree of postoperative ileus, a physiological arrest of GI transit in response to surgical stress and intestinal manipulation. Neostigmine can increase motility only if acetylcholine release and smooth muscle function are relatively preserved, while postoperative ileus induces the activation of presynaptic noradrenergic receptors and impairs the functionality of the enteric nervous system and the sympathetic nerves [19,20]. This could have determined the absence of the expected effects on intestinal and gastric motility.

Moreover, in the study by Yağan, neostigmine doses were higher than those used in our study [13], and the correlation between the neostigmine dose and PONV is now considered a key factor to control the symptoms [9].

Two scales were employed as awakening quality indicators: MMSt and OASS. The MMSt was considered to assess cognitive impairment because it is a rapid and simple to perform test that provides accurate measurements of cognitive status both in subjects with normal functions and in subjects with cognitive alterations [21], and its use to assess subtle changes in cognitive function after anesthesia is often reported [22].

Our results have unexpectedly shown a significant increase of the average value of MMSt in the considered time frames. The OASS mean value also significantly increased in the S group until 1 h after surgery.

The reversal action of sugammadex is based on the structure of cyclodextrins, consisting of a lipophilic central cavity able to encapsulate the steroid rings of the rocuronium molecule, forming an inactive complex that is no longer able to interact with the neuromuscular junction [23]. Based on its structural characteristics, the fact that the sugammadex molecule or the sugammadex/rocuronium complex could interact in any way with the anesthetic drugs or with the cholinergic system was excluded [24]. The apparent rapid awakening at a cognitive level, that some other authors and we have detected [25,26], could be explained in the light of the so-called Afferentation Theory [27], for which general activation of muscle receptors can induce a massive cerebral stimulation of the monoaminergic wakefulness centers. It is also known as the Spindle Theory [23], since it has been postulated that tension and stretch receptors in muscle spindles may be the terminations that transmit static and dynamic variations to the encephalon, acting on various cortical and mesencephalic areas. However, some studies have not been able to demonstrate changes in the depth of anesthesia after sugammadex administration [28], thus the results of studies regarding sugammadex's impact on recovery from general anesthesia remain conflicting and insufficient [29].

In the past, many studies demonstrated an existing relationship between the structure of cyclodextrins and neuroprotection: statins and cyclodextrins, influence the transmission of neural signals, interfering with the production of inflammatory molecules [30]. Ultimately, one could speculate that sugammadex gives an additional effect by interacting with the lipid molecules of the neuronal membrane, reducing exocytosis. This protective effect could be more readily detectable in a surgery, such as robotic cystectomy, which requires more than 2 h in steep Trendelenburg and alterations of cerebrovascular circulation due to prolonged pneumoperitoneum [10]. In the future, it could be interesting to analyze if the use of sugammadex can be optimized, employing it in elderly populations or in surgeries that require high abdominal pressure or extreme conditions.

A limit of our study mainly regards the same limitations related to the neurophysiological tests administered in the postoperative period. These tests may be subject to the learning effect bias and to the variability in the sessions following the preoperative one, considered baseline, and from one session to another. We tried to minimize this variability by administering the test in the same environment, with no external distractions, and patients who needed extra doses of opioids for pain were excluded.

5. Conclusions

In conclusion, our results were not able to demonstrate a significant decrease of the PONV or a more rapid ROI after sugammadex administration versus neostigmine use. We observed a significant increase in MMSt values, suggesting improved quality of awakening with the use of sugammadex in patients undergoing robotic radical cystectomy. Regarding OASS observations in both groups, we obtained higher values in the group receiving sugammadex. Further studies on elderly populations and different types of surgery will be needed in the future, especially with the aim to provide a comprehensive ERAS pathway for cystectomy based on the available evidence.

Author Contributions: Conceptualization, C.C. and E.F.; methodology, C.C.; formal analysis, C.C.; investigation, C.C., M.C. and G.T. (Giulia Torregiani); data curation, M.E.M., A.S.d.U., A.Z., G.T. (Gabriele Tuderti) and G.S.; writing—original draft preparation, C.C.; writing—review and editing, C.C., M.C. and G.T. (Giulia Torregiani); supervision, E.F.

Funding: This research received no external funding.

Acknowledgments: Editorial assistance was provided by Luca Giacomelli and Aashni Shah (Polistudium).

Conflicts of Interest: The authors declare no conflict of interest.

References

1. Leow, J.J.; Chang, S.L.; Meyer, C.P.; Wang, Y.; Hanske, J.; Sammon, J.D.; Cole, A.P.; Preston, M.A.; Dasgupta, P.; Menon, M.; et al. Robot-assisted Versus Open Radical Prostatectomy: A Contemporary Analysis of an All-payer Discharge Database. *Eur. Urol.* **2016**, *70*, 837–845. [CrossRef]
2. Trentman, T.L.; Fassett, S.L.; McGirr, D.; Anderson, B.; Chang, Y.H.H.; Nateras, R.N.; Castle, E.P.; Rosenfeld, D.M. Comparison of anesthetic management and outcomes of robot-assisted versus open radical cystectomy. *J. Robot. Surg.* **2013**, *7*, 273–279. [CrossRef]
3. Oksar, M.; Akbulut, Z.; Ocal, H.; Balbay, M.D.; Kanbak, O. Anesthetic considerations for robotic cystectomy: A prospective study. *Braz. J. Anesthesiol.* **2014**, *64*, 109–115. [CrossRef]
4. Cockcroft, J.O.; Berry, C.B.; McGrath, J.S.; Daugherty, M.O. Anesthesia for Major Urologic Surgery. *Anesthesiol. Clin.* **2015**, *33*, 165–172. [CrossRef]
5. Martini, C.H.; Boon, M.; Bevers, R.F.; Aarts, L.P.; Dahan, A. Evaluation of Surgical Conditions During Laparoscopic Surgery in Patients with Moderate vs. Deep Neuromuscular Block. *Surv. Anesthesiol.* **2014**, *58*, 222–223. [CrossRef]

6. Boon, M.; Martini, C.H.; Aarts, L.P.; Bevers, R.F.; Dahan, A. Effect of variations in depth of neuromuscular blockade on rating of surgical conditions by surgeon and anesthesiologist in patients undergoing laparoscopic renal or prostatic surgery (BLISS trial): Study protocol for a randomized controlled trial. *Trials* **2013**, *14*, 63. [CrossRef]
7. Geldner, G.; Niskanen, M.; Laurila, P.; Mizikov, V.; Hübler, M.; Beck, G.; Rietbergen, H.; Nicolayenko, E. A randomized controlled trial comparing sugammadex and neostigmine at different depths of neuromuscular blockade in patients undergoing laparoscopic surgery. *Anaesthesia* **2012**, *67*, 991–998. [CrossRef]
8. Paton, F.; Paulden, M.; Chambers, D.; Heirs, M.; Duffy, S.; Hunter, J.M.; Sculpher, M.; Woolacott, N. Sugammadex compared with neostigmine/glycopyrrolate for routine reversal of neuromuscular block: A systematic review and economic evaluation. *Br. J. Anaesth.* **2010**, *105*, 558–567. [CrossRef]
9. Luo, J.; Chen, S.; Min, S.; Peng, L. Reevaluation and update on efficacy and safety of neostigmine for reversal of neuromuscular blockade. *Ther. Clin. Risk Manag.* **2018**, *14*, 2397–2406. [CrossRef]
10. Kamine, T.H.; Papavassiliou, E.; Schneider, B.E. Effect of Abdominal Insufflation for Laparoscopy on Intracranial Pressure. *JAMA Surg.* **2014**, *149*, 380. [CrossRef]
11. Cerantola, Y.; Valerio, M.; Persson, B.; Jichlinski, P.; Ljungqvist, O.; Hübner, M.; Kassouf, W.; Müller, S.; Baldini, G.; Carli, F.; et al. Guidelines for perioperative care after radical cystectomy for bladder cancer: Enhanced Recovery After Surgery (ERAS®) society recommendations. *Clin. Nutr.* **2013**, *32*, 879–887. [CrossRef]
12. Simone, G.; Papalia, R.; Misuraca, L.; Tuderti, G.; Minisola, F.; Ferriero, M.; Vallati, G.E.; Guaglianone, S.; Gallucci, M. Robotic Intracorporeal Padua Ileal Bladder: Surgical Technique, Perioperative, Oncologic and Functional Outcomes. *Eur. Urol.* **2018**, *73*, 934–940. [CrossRef]
13. Yağan, Ö.; Taş, N.; Mutlu, T.; Hancı, V.; Hanci, V. Comparison of the effects of sugammadex and neostigmine on postoperative nausea and vomiting. *Braz. J. Anesthesiol.* **2017**, *67*, 147–152.
14. Løvstad, R.Z.; Thagaard, K.S.; Berner, N.S.; Raeder, J.C. Neostigmine 50 microg kg(−1) with glycopyrrolate increases postoperative nausea in women after laparoscopic gynecological surgery. *Acta Anaesthesiol. Scand.* **2001**, *45*, 495–500. [CrossRef]
15. Law, N.-M.; Bharucha, A.E.; Undale, A.S.; Zinsmeister, A.R. Cholinergic stimulation enhances colonic motor activity, transit, and sensation in humans. *Am. J. Physiol. Gastrointest. Liver Physiol.* **2001**, *281*, G1228–G1237. [CrossRef]
16. Lassen, K.; Soop, M.; Nygren, J.; Cox, P.B.W.; Hendry, P.O.; Spies, C.; von Meyenfeldt, M.F.; Fearon, K.C.; Revhaug, A.; Norderval, S.; et al. Enhanced Recovery After Surgery (ERAS) Group. Consensus review of optimal perioperative care in colorectal surgery: Enhanced Recovery After Surgery (ERAS) Group recommendations. *Arch. Surg.* **2009**, *144*, 961–969. [CrossRef]
17. Paech, M.J.; Kaye, R.; Baber, C.; Nathan, E.A. Recovery characteristics of patients receiving either sugammadex or neostigmine and glycopyrrolate for reversal of neuromuscular block: A randomised controlled trial. *Anaesthesia* **2018**, *73*, 340–347. [CrossRef]
18. Koyuncu, O.; Turhanoglu, S.; Akkurt, C.O.; Karcıoğlu, M.; Ozkan, M.; Ozer, C.; Sessler, D.I.; Turan, A. Comparison of sugammadex and conventional reversal on postoperative nausea and vomiting: A randomized, blinded trial. *J. Clin. Anesth.* **2015**, *27*, 51–56. [CrossRef]
19. Goetz, B.; Benhaqi, P.; Müller, M.H.; Kreis, M.E.; Kasparek, M.S. Changes in beta-adrenergic neurotransmission during postoperative ileus in rat circular jejunal muscle. *Neurogastroenterol. Motil.* **2013**, *25*, 154-e84. [CrossRef]
20. Neunlist, M.; Rolli-Derkinderen, M.; Latorre, R.; Van Landeghem, L.; Coron, E.; Derkinderen, P.; De Giorgio, R. Enteric Glial Cells: Recent Developments and Future Directions. *Gastroenterology* **2014**, *147*, 1230–1237. [CrossRef]
21. Rasmussen, L.S.; Larsen, K.; Houx, P.; Skovgaard, L.T.; Hanning, C.D.; Moller, J.T. The assessment of postoperative cognitive function. *Acta Anaesthesiol. Scand.* **2001**, *45*, 275–289. [CrossRef] [PubMed]
22. KUŞKU, A.; Demir, G.; Çukurova, Z.; Eren, G.; Hergünsel, O. Monitorization of the effects of spinal anaesthesia on cerebral oxygen saturation in elder patients using near-infrared spectroscopy. *Braz. J. Anesthesiol.* **2014**, *64*, 241–246. [PubMed]
23. Adam, J.M.; Bennett, D.J.; Bom, A.; Clark, J.K.; Feilden, H.; Hutchinson, E.J.; Palin, R.; Prosser, A.; Rees, D.C.; Rosair, G.M.; et al. Cyclodextrin-Derived Host Molecules as Reversal Agents for the Neuromuscular Blocker Rocuronium Bromide: Synthesis and Structure-Activity Relationships. *J. Med. Chem.* **2002**, *45*, 1806–1816. [CrossRef] [PubMed]

24. Sparr, H.J.; Vermeyen, K.M.; Beaufort, A.M.; Rietbergen, H.; Proost, J.H.; Saldien, V.; Velik-Salchner, C.; Wierda, J.M. Early reversal of profound rocuronium-induced neuromuscular blockade by sugammadex in a randomized multicenter study: Efficacy, safety, and pharmacokinetics. *Anesthesiology* **2007**, *106*, 935–943. [CrossRef]
25. Amorim, P.; Lagarto, F.; Gomes, B.; Esteves, S.; Bismarck, J.; Rodrigues, N.; Nogueira, M. Neostigmine vs. sugammadex: Observational cohort study comparing the quality of recovery using the Postoperative Quality Recovery Scale. *Acta Anaesthesiol. Scand.* **2014**, *58*, 1101–1110. [CrossRef]
26. Chazot, T.; Dumont, G.; Le Guen, M.; Hausser-Hauw, C.; Liu, N.; Fischler, M. Sugammadex administration results in arousal from intravenous anaesthesia: A clinical and electroencephalographic observation. *Br. J. Anaesth.* **2011**, *106*, 914–916. [CrossRef]
27. Lanier, W.L.; Laizzo, P.A.; Milde, J.H.; Sharbrough, F.W. The Cerebral and Systemic Effects of Movement in Response to a Noxious Stimulus in Lightly Anesthetized Dogs Possible Modulation of Cerebral Function by Muscle Afferents. *Anesthesiology* **1994**, *80*, 392–401. [CrossRef]
28. Illman, H.; Antila, H.; Olkkola, K.T. Reversal of neuromuscular blockade by sugammadex does not affect EEG derived indices of depth of anesthesia. *J. Clin. Monit. Comput.* **2010**, *24*, 371–376. [CrossRef]
29. Sadhasivam, S.; Ganesh, A.; Robison, A.; Kaye, R.; Watcha, M.F. Validation of the Bispectral Index Monitor for Measuring the Depth of Sedation in Children. *Anesth. Analg.* **2006**, *102*, 383–388. [CrossRef]
30. Abulrob, A.; Tauskela, J.S.; Mealing, G.; Brunette, E.; Faid, K.; Stanimirovic, D. Protection by cholesterol-extracting cyclodextrins: A role for N-methyl-d-aspartate receptor redistribution. *J. Neurochem.* **2005**, *92*, 1477–1486. [CrossRef]

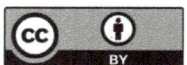

© 2019 by the authors. Licensee MDPI, Basel, Switzerland. This article is an open access article distributed under the terms and conditions of the Creative Commons Attribution (CC BY) license (http://creativecommons.org/licenses/by/4.0/).

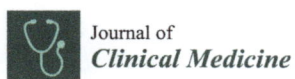

Article

Do Younger Patients with Muscle-Invasive Bladder Cancer have Better Outcomes?

Florian Janisch [1,2], Hang Yu [1], Malte W. Vetterlein [1], Roland Dahlem [1], Oliver Engel [1], Margit Fisch [1], Shahrokh F. Shariat [2,3,4,5,6,7], Armin Soave [1] and Michael Rink [1,*]

1. Department of Urology, Medical University of Hamburg, Martinistraße 52, 20246 Hamburg, Germany; drfjanisch@gmail.com (F.J.); yuhang.seu@outlook.com (H.Y.); malte.vetterlein@googlemail.com (M.W.V.); r.dahlem@uke.de (R.D.); o.engel@uke.de (O.E.); m.fisch@uke.de (M.F.); armin.soave@googlemail.com (A.S.)
2. Department of Urology, Medical University of Vienna, Währinger Gürtel 18-20, 1090 Vienna, Austria; sfshariat@gmail.com
3. Institute for Urology and Reproductive Health, Sechenov University, Bolshaya Pirogovskaya str. 2-4, 119991 Moscow, Russia
4. Department of Urology, Weill Cornell Medical School, 1300 York Avenue, New York, NY 10065, USA
5. Department of Urology, University of Texas Southwestern Medical Center, 5323 Harry Hines Blvd, Dallas, TX 75390, USA
6. Karl Landsteiner Institute of Urology and Andrology, Franziskanergasse 4, a 3100 St. Poelten, Austria
7. Department of Urology, Second Faculty of Medicine, Charles University, Ovocný trh 5, Prague 1-116 36, Czech Republic
* Correspondence: m.rink@uke.de; Tel.: +49-40-7410-53442; Fax: +49-40-7410-52444

Received: 12 August 2019; Accepted: 11 September 2019; Published: 13 September 2019

Abstract: Urothelial cancer of the bladder (UCB) is usually a disease of the elderly. The influence of age on oncological outcomes remains controversial. This study aims to investigate the impact of age on UCB outcomes in Europe focusing particularly on young and very young patients. We collected data of 669 UCB patients treated with RC at our tertiary care center. We used various categorical stratifications as well as continuous age to investigate the association of age and tumor biology as well as endpoints with descriptive statistics and Cox regression. The median age was 67 years and the mean follow-up was 52 months. Eight patients (1.2%) were ≤40 years old and 39 patients (5.8%) were aged 41–50 years, respectively. In multivariable analysis, higher continuous age and age above the median were independent predictors for disease recurrence, and cancer-specific and overall mortality (all p-values ≤ 0.018). In addition, patients with age in the oldest tertile group had inferior cancer-specific and overall survival rates compared to their younger counterparts. Young (40–50 years) and very young (≤40 years) patients had reduced hazards for all endpoints, which, however, were not statistically significant. Age remains an independent determinant for survival after RC. Young adults did, however, not have superior outcomes in our analyses. Quality of life and complications are endpoints that need further evaluation in patients undergoing RC.

Keywords: bladder cancer; age; urothelial carcinoma; radical cystectomy; outcome; survival

1. Introduction

With an incidence of over 80,000 new cases and over 17,000 deaths estimated to occur in 2019 in the United States alone, urothelial cancer of the bladder (UCB) is the second leading genitourinary malignancy and a potentially lethal disease [1]. Compared with other malignancies, UCB is usually a disease of the elderly with a peak incidence among those in their 70s [2,3]. In fact, in general there is an increasing life expectancy in the US and Europe and in consequence, a potential further rise in UCB diagnoses is expected in the next few decades [4,5]. Ageing trends are of major scientific and clinical importance in any cancer including UCB, as the optimal management has great impact for each individuum and the public health system in general, especially in an expensive disease as UCB [6].

Despite the overwhelming incidence in elderly patients, UCB does also occur in a non-negligible number of young patients [3]. While the development of UCB in the elderly has been suggested to be driven by a cumulative lifetime exposure to environmentally, occupationally, or individually acquired carcinogens (e.g., smoking) [7–9], the factors for UCB in young patients remain rather inconclusive. Not only the diagnosis of UCB, particularly the need of RC with all its negative effects on quality of life has a significant impact on the psyche and more, especially in the younger. RC is more frequently offered in younger patients, due to their longer life expectancy, lower frailty resulting in lower adverse events and the superiority in survival outcomes of early compared to delayed RC [10]. Recent reports suggest superior UCB-specific outcomes in young and adolescent patients (15–39 years) [11].

The impact of patient age on oncological outcomes remains controversial and regional variabilities may be present that need to be considered in patient counselling and treatment planning. The aim of this study was to evaluate the impact of age on UCB outcomes after RC in a consecutive cohort of European patients, particularly focusing on the young and very young. We hypothesized that younger patients may have better oncologic outcomes as their disease may be earlier in their natural history and different as it may not have a large mutational burden.

2. Material and Methods

2.1. Patient Population

We retrospectively reviewed the medical records of 789 consecutive patients treated with RC and bilateral pelvic lymphadenectomy for UCB between 1996 and 2011 at our institution. Guideline adherent indications for RC were muscle invasive UCB or recurrent Ta, T1, or carcinoma in situ (CIS) refractory to transurethral resection of the bladder (TURB) with or without intravesical chemo- or immunotherapy. As neoadjuvant chemotherapy may be more frequently administered in younger patients, implementing an inherent bias of natural UCB history in age analyses, these patients were excluded upfront ($n = 8$). Moreover, 75 patients were excluded because of missing variables or follow-up, 30 patients with RC for non-malignant indication for RC, and seven patients with advanced, bladder infiltrating prostate cancer. In total, 669 patients remained for analyses. Overall, 147 patients (20.0%) received adjuvant chemotherapy (95% platinum-based) at the clinicians' discretion in accordance with the guidelines at the time. The study was approved by the local ethics committee.

2.2. Follow-Up Regimen

Follow-up strategy has been previously reported in detail [12,13]. In brief, patients were generally seen every three to four months for the first year after surgery, every six months from the second to fifth year, and annually thereafter. Follow-up included a history, physical examination and serum chemistry evaluation. Diagnostic imaging of the abdomen including the urinary tract and chest radiography were performed at least annually or when clinically indicated. Additional radiographic evaluations were performed when clinically indicated.

2.3. Statistical Analysis

Statistical analyses included demographic data on patients' age, ethnicity, gender, ASA status, pathologic tumor stage and grade, concomitant CIS, lymph node status, margin status, lymphovascular invasion, and adjuvant chemotherapy, respectively.

The co-primary endpoints were recurrence-free survival (RFS), cancer-specific survival (CSS), and overall survival (OS), respectively. Disease recurrence was defined as local failure in the operative site, regional lymph nodes, or distant metastasis. Upper tract urothelial carcinoma was considered a metachronous tumor and not disease recurrence. Patients who did not experience disease recurrence were censored at time of last follow-up for recurrence-free survival analysis. Cancer-specific mortality was defined as death from UCB. The cause of death was determined by the treating physician, by chart review corroborated by death certificates, or by death certificates alone [14]. Perioperative mortality (i.e., death within 30 days of surgery) was censored at time of death for UCB-specific survival analyses.

Age was analyzed as a continuous variable, with a cut-off at median and tertiles, and using the cut-offs of 50 years. (dichotomized) and ≤40, 41–50, and >50 years (three categories), respectively. The different analytic approaches were used to optimally approach the definition of young age. There is no clear determination for UCB patients treated with RC in the urologic literature defining a patient as 'young' or 'very young'. However, there is a consensus among oncological experts that patients <50 years. are usually defined as 'young' and patients <40 years. defined as 'very young' [15]. Using median and tertiles as cut-off, we investigated the effects of age in our study population with homogenous sample distributions. Utilization of the dichotomized cut-off of 50 years. was based on previous reports that indicated superior survival outcomes in patients <50 years. The tri-categorical analyses uses cut-offs of <40 years and <50 years following predefined ranges indicated by the NCI in 2006 [15]. In addition, study results indicate significant outcome differences, suggesting these strata represent an ideal standard [11].

The Kolmogorov–Smirnov test was used to assess the normal distribution of variables. The Fisher's exact test and the chi-square test were used to evaluate the association between categorical variables. Differences in variables with a continuous distribution across categories were assessed using the Mann–Whitney U test (two categories) and Kruskal–Wallis test (three and more categories). Actuarial method was used to estimate RFS, CSS, and OS probabilities and the differences were assessed with the log rank test. Kaplan–Meier estimates were used to graphically display survival functions. Univariable and multivariable Cox regression models addressed time-to-event endpoint analyses. In all models, proportional hazards assumptions were systematically verified using the Grambsch–Therneau residual-based test. Multicollinearity was assessed with the variance inflation factor to test for possible confounding between relevant covariates. All reported p-values were two-sided, and statistical significance was set at $p < 0.05$. All statistical tests were performed with IBM SPSS Statistics 25 (IBM Corp., Armonk, NY, USA).

3. Results

3.1. Association of Age with Clinical–Pathological Characteristics

The median age of the study cohort was 67 years (interquartile range [IQR]: 59; 73), and 520 (78%) of the patients were male. In total, 622 patients (93.0%) were older than 50 years. Of those being <50 years, 39 patients (5.8%) were aged 41–50 years and 8 patients (1.2%) were younger than 40 years. Tertiles for age were ≤59 years (first tertile), 60–72 years (second tertile), and ≥73 years (third tertile), respectively. The descriptive clinicopathologic characteristics of the study cohort are presented in Table 1.

Table 1. Descriptive characteristics stratified by dichotomy age groups of 669 UCB patients treated with radical cystectomy

	All	Young (≤50)		Elderly (≥51)	p-Value	p-Value
		≤40	41–50	≥51	≤50 vs. ≥51	≤40 vs. 41–50 vs. ≥51
Patients, n	669	8	39	622	-	-
Gender (%)					0.85	0.98
Male	520 (77.7)	6 (75.0)	30 (76.9)	484 (77.8)		
Female	149 (22.3)	2 (25.0)	9 (23.1)	138 (22.2)		
ASA (%)					<0.001	<0.001
1	52 (7.8)	4 (50.0)	7 (18.0)	41 (6.6)		
2	386 (57.7)	3 (37.5)	27 (69.2)	356 (57.2)		
3	225 (33.6)	1 (12.5)	3 (7.7)	221 (35.5)		
4	6 (0.9)	0 (0)	2 (5.1)	4 (0.7)		
Pathological Tumor Stage (%)					0.92	0.34
pT0	73 (10.9)	3 (37.5)	4 (10.3)	66 (10.6)		

Table 1. Cont.

	All	Young (≤50)		Elderly (≥51)	p-Value	p-Value
		≤40	41–50	≥51	≤50 vs. ≥51	≤40 vs. 41–50 vs. ≥51
pTa	26 (3.9)	0 (0)	1 (2.6)	25 (4.0)		
pTis	66 (9.9)	0 (0)	3 (7.7)	63 (10.1)		
pT1	74 (11.1)	1 (12.5)	4 (10.3)	69 (11.1)		
pT2	132 (19.7)	0 (0)	10 (25.6)	122 (19.6)		
pT3	182 (27.2)	4 (50.0)	8 (20.5)	170 (27.3)		
pT4	116 (17.3)	0 (0)	9 (23.1)	107 (17.2)		
Pathological Tumor Grade (%)					0.58	0.42
No grading (pT0)	73 (10.9)	3 (37.5)	4 (10.3)	66 (10.6)		
G2	65 (9.7)	1 (12.5)	6 (15.4)	58 (9.3)		
G3	531 (79.4)	4 (50.0)	29 (74.3)	498 (80.1)		
Concomitant carcinoma in situ (%)					0.051	0.12
Absent	424 (63.4)	7 (87.5)	29 (74.4)	388 (62.4)		
Present	245 (36.6)	1 (12.5)	10 (25.6)	234 (37.6)		
Lymph node status (%)					0.91	0.58
pN0	479 (71.6)	7 (87.5)	27 (69.2)	445 (71.5)		
pN+	190 (28.4)	1 (12.5)	12 (30.8)	177 (28.5)		
Margin status (%)					0.94	0.99
R0	586 (87.6)	7 (87.5)	34 (87.2)	545 (87.6)		
R+	83 (12.4)	1 (12.5)	5 (12.8)	77 (12.4)		
Lymphovascular invasion (%)					0.52	0.62
L0	455 (68.0)	6 (75)	24 (61.5)	425 (68.3)		
L1	214 (32.0)	2 (25)	15 (38.5)	197 (31.7)		
Adjuvant Chemotherapy (%)					0.089	0.21
No	522 (78.0)	6 (75.0)	26 (66.7)	490 (78.8)		
Yes	147 (22.0)	2 (25.0)	13 (33.3)	132 (21.2)		

Comparing patients under and over 50, older patients presented with a significantly higher ASA score ($p < 0.001$). ASA scores increased significantly from patients ≤40 years to patients aged 41–50 and to ≥50 years ($p < 0.001$). There were no statistically significant differences in any other clinical–pathological variables irrespective of the stratification used.

3.2. Association of Age with Disease Recurrence and Survival Outcomes

The median follow-up was 52 months (IQR: 17; 78). During the follow-up period, 192 patients (32.4%) experienced disease recurrence, 175 patients (28.0%) died of UCB, and 257 patients (42.1%) died of any cause. The actuarial recurrence-free survival estimates at 2- and 5-years after RC were 64 ± 2% and 59 ± 2%, respectively. The actuarial cancer-specific survival estimates at 2- and 5-years after RC were 71 ± 2% and 61 ± 3%, respectively. The actuarial overall-specific survival estimates at 2- and 5-years after RC were 62 ± 2% and 50 ± 2%, respectively.

In the Kaplan–Meier analyses, no statistically significant difference was observed in recurrence-free survival ($p = 0.49$; Figure 1A), cancer-specific survival ($p = 0.78$; Figure 1C), and overall survival ($p = 0.67$; Figure 1E) between patients younger than 50 years, and those 50 and above. In categorical age group analyses, there was also no statistically significant difference in recurrence-free survival, cancer-specific survival and overall survival ($p > 0.05$ for all; Figure 1B,D,F) between patients 50 years and above, those between 41–50 years and those 40 and younger.

3.3. Risk Factor Analyses for Disease Recurrence and Survival Outcomes

All variables tested on multicollinearity had an VIF in the range of 1.1–2.9, indicating that no multicollinearity is present between factors included in the cox regression model. The results of univariable Cox regression analyses for different age stratifications are presented in Table 2. Higher continuous age was significantly associated with inferior recurrence-free (Hazard ratio (HR): 1.017; 95%CI: 1.002–1.032; $p = 0.029$), cancer-specific (HR: 1.023; 95%CI: 1.007–1.039; $p = 0.005$), and overall survival (HR: 1.030; 95%CI: 1.016–1.044; $p < 0.001$). In addition, patients older than the median (all $p \leq 0.01$) and patients in the highest age tertile compared to patients in the second tertile (all $p \leq 0.008$) were significantly associated with inferior outcomes for all three endpoints. Analyses according to all age categories (i.e., $\leq$50 vs $>$50; $\leq$40 vs. 41–50 vs. $>$50, tertiles) revealed that patients in higher age categories were not associated with a higher risk for all endpoints (all $p > 0.05$).

The results of multivariable Cox regression analyses that adjusted for standard UCB clinic-pathological parameters (Table 3) showed that higher continuous age (RFS HR: 1.019; $p = 0.018$; CSS HR: 1.025; $p = 0.004$, and OS HR: 1.030; $p < 0.001$), age above the median of our cohort (RFS HR: 1.472; $p = 0.014$; CSS HR: 1.553; $p = 0.008$; and OS HR: 1.596; $p = 0.001$) and age in the third tertile ($\geq$73 years) compared to the second age tertile (60–72 years) (RFS HR: 1.862; $p = 0.005$; CSS HR: 2.085; $p = 0.001$; OS HR: 2.256; $p < 0.001$) were all independently associated with worse outcomes for all three endpoints. In addition, CSS and OS of patients in the third tertile were also inferior compared to the outcomes of patients in the first age tertile ($\leq$59 years) (CSS HR: 1.545; $p \leq 0.034$; OS HR 1.728; $p = 0.002$).

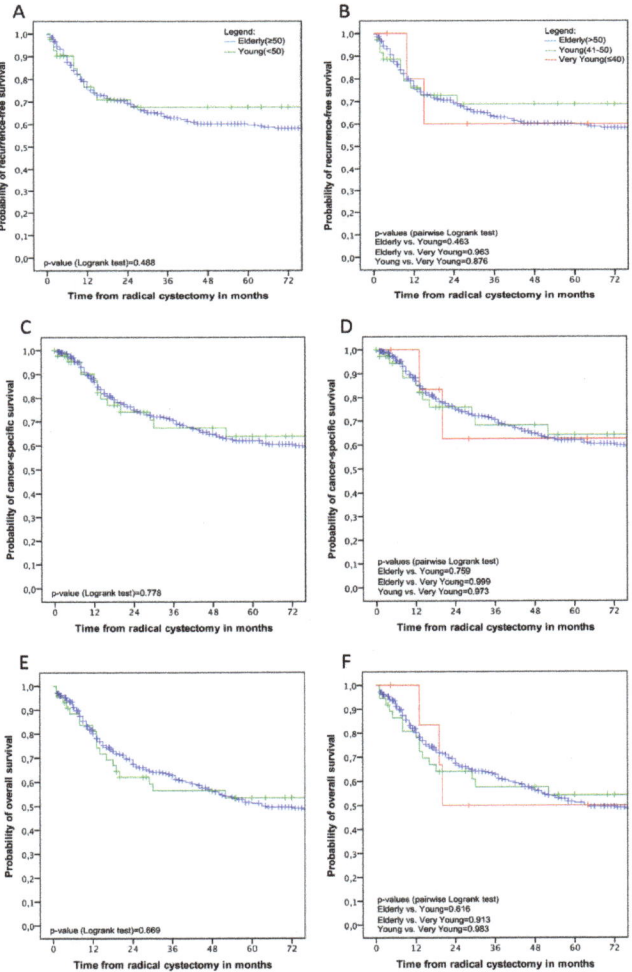

Figure 1. Kaplan–Meier estimates of stratified age groups of elderly ($\geq$50 years.) and young patients (<50 years.) (**A,C,E**), and stratified in three age groups of elderly (>50 years.) young (41–50 years.) and very young ($\leq$40 years.) patients (**B,D,F**) for recurrence-free, cancer-specific, and overall survival, respectively.

Table 2. Univariable cox regression analysis of variable age stratifications predicting recurrence-free survival, cancer-specific survival and overall survival of 669 patients with UCB treated with radical cystectomy.

Age Stratifications	RFS			CSS			OS		
	HR	95%CI	p-Value	HR	95%CI	p-Value	HR	95%CI	p-Value
Continuous age	1.017	1.002–1.032	0.029	1.023	1.007–1.039	0.005	1.030	1.016–1.044	<0.001
Median Age	1.454	1.095–1.932	0.010	1.550	1.150–2.088	0.004	1.663	1.299–2.129	<0.001
Age ≤50 vs. >50	1.227	0.684–2.202	0.49	1.084	0.616–1.909	0.78	1.107	0.693–1.767	0.67
Age (three categories)									
≤40 vs. >50	0.818	0.179–3.733	0.80	0.910	0.202–4.111	0.90	0.832	0.242–2.858	0.77
41–50 vs. >50	1.035	0.257–4.170	0.96	1.001	0.248–4.038	0.99	0.946	0.303–2.955	0.92
Age (Tertiles)									
first vs. third tertile	1.242	0.861–1.793	0.25	1.364	0.926–2.008	0.12	1.576	1.137–2.185	0.006
second vs. third tertile	1.699	1.151–2.507	0.008	1.931	1.278–2.917	0.002	2.194	1.546–3.112	<0.001

Abbreviations: RFS = recurrence free survival; CSS = cancer specific survival; OS = overall survival; HR = hazard ratio; CI = confidence interval; UCB = urothelial carcinoma of the bladder.

Table 3. Multivariable cox regression analysis of the effect of age on predicting recurrence-free survival, cancer-specific survival and overall survival of 669 patients with UCB and treated with radical cystectomy.

Age Stratifications	RFS			CSS			OS		
	HR	95%CI	p-Value	HR	95%CI	p-Value	HR	95%CI	p-Value
Continuous Age	1.019	1.003–1.035	0.018	1.025	1.008–1.042	0.004	1.030	1.016–1.045	0.000
Median age	1.472	1.081–2.005	0.014	1.553	1.124–2.146	0.008	1.596	1.225–2.080	0.001
Age (Tertiles)									
first vs. third tertile	1.339	0.914–1.962	0.13	1.545	1.033–2.312	0.034	1.728	1.230–2.428	0.002
second vs. third tertile	1.862	1.211–2.864	0.005	2.085	1.328–3.276	0.001	2.256	1.541–3.304	<0.001

All multivariable analyses were adjusted for the following co-variables: gender, ASA score, pathological tumor stage, pathological tumor grade, concomitant carcinoma in situ, lymph node status, margin status, lymphovascular invasion, and adjuvant chemotherapy. Abbreviations: RFS = recurrence free survival; CSS = cancer specific survival; OS = overall survival; HR = hazard ratio; CI = confidence interval; UCB = urothelial carcinoma of the bladder.

4. Discussion

We found that young patients did not present with more favorable tumor biological features compared to their older counterparts. In addition, we did not find significantly superior survival outcomes for all three endpoints in favor of young patients. Therefore, we reject our hypothesis that young UCB patients with MIBC have better outcomes post-RC than the normal MIBC patient. This is in contrast to previous studies that reported better oncological outcomes in younger UCB populations [11,16,17]. Differences in results between our study and previous reports may be explained by different definition of young age, diverse race/ethnicity or distinct socioeconomic status, etc. [18]. Indeed, we found that higher continuous age and other strata defining patients as elderly were independently associated with inferior survival outcomes. Thus, while one end of the age spectrum does not better, the other end of the spectrum seems to have worse oncologic outcomes. Undeniably, this underscores the validity of our UCB cohort as these findings are in line with those of large, multicentric UCB series [19,20].

The relationship between age and prognosis of UCB remains controversial. In fact, there is no clear definition when a UCB patient is defined to be very young, young, old, or very old. A recent large US study reported that adolescents and young UCB patients (ages 15–39) [11] had superior cancer-specific and overall survival compared to their older counterparts. In another study, patients were stratified using a cut-off of 50 years with superior cancer-specific and overall survival in the younger group [16]. In our study we, therefore, used variable age stratifications and cut-offs to reflect the most comprehensive picture on the impact of age across a wide spectrum of definitions and results. Indeed, using this comprehensive approach, we only found differences in categorized outcome analyses when using the median age or age tertiles of our cohort. Of importance, the median age in our cohort was 67 years and the upper age tertile included patients above 73 years. Thus, despite depicting a statistical significance compared to 'younger patients' in our cohort, our data did not demonstrate superior outcomes in those patients usually defined to be young or very young.

From the biological rationale it intuitively seems reasonable that older patients may experience inferior outcomes. With increasing age, exposure to several environmental, occupational, and individually amenable (e.g., smoking) stressors accumulate over time [7,21,22]. In addition, especially elderly men often experience obstructive lower urinary tract symptoms with incomplete bladder drainage. In consequence, the potentially prolonged contact time to carcinogens excreted in the urine may induce accumulation of cellular events that can lead to neoplastic transformation and subsequently UCB development [20]. Moreover, younger patients tend to be healthier in general, with mostly good immunity and nutrition status, as well as fewer co-morbidities to tolerate the complications of cancers or treatment.

From a clinical perspective, our results are important, as recent studies found very young UCB patients to have a lower hazard of cancer-specific mortality compared to their older counterparts [11], suggesting that organ-sparing approaches may be a viable option in young patients [23–25]. Especially the prospect of incontinence, impotence and/or infertility due to radical cystectomy may lead to delay of therapy or a switch of strategy to a bladder sparing, multimodal approach. However, younger patients are more reluctant to undergo necessary diagnostics and treatments or comply with strict follow-up schedules, possibly affecting outcomes [26]. In agreement with our results, other investigators also found either no difference [27] or even worse outcomes, due to a higher rate of metastases [28], in patients ≤40 years. A potential reason for the disparity in findings of various studies including ours may be due to difference in ethnicities, regional varieties in treatment, different socioeconomic backgrounds, and other factors that we could not all adjust for in our analyses. However, despite our findings not providing a final answer on the influence of a very young age on UCB outcomes treated with RC, our results do generate hypotheses that warrant further investigation of this association in larger, multi-institutional, ideally prospective studies. Indeed, our findings support the surgical approach of radical cystectomy also in young and very-young patients, as our findings underscore the aggressive nature of UCB and no age-group had superior survival outcomes.

Certainly, the reconstruction which affects quality of life and perceived self-image should be adopted to patients' preferences, and general and specific health factors [29].

Our study is not devoid of limitations. First and foremost, the retrospective and single-center nature may inevitably introduce some selection bias. Despite this being a large monocentric cohort of consecutive patients, the overall sample size is still limited, especially in the subgroup of very young patients. Nevertheless, we feel that our study still provides a representative insight on age-dependent prognostic outcomes for Europe. All patients in our study were Caucasians, which should be considered since ethnicity may influence survival in UCB [30,31]. We were unable to collect and adjust analyses for several predisposing risk factors of UCB, including smoking, occupational exposure, family history, insurance status, immunity or nutrition status, adjuvant therapies, or socio-economic factors that also may influence tumor biology or outcomes [22,32,33]. In addition, laboratory and molecular data was not available. However, from the clinical perspective, the latter information is usually not available in daily routine for patient counselling. Age in general does represent a competing risk for death particularly since older patients have a greater frailty and UCB patients often harbor important comorbidities [34–36]. However, due to sample size limitations, we were unable to perform competing-risk analyses. Consequently, a contemporary, European multicenter approach would be warranted to shed further insight on this relevant topic.

5. Conclusions

In conclusion, we found that young age at time of MIBC diagnosis does not result in better outcomes compared to typical age after RC. Higher age, however, remains an important prognostic factor for cancer-related endpoints in UCB and thus needs to be incorporated in therapeutic considerations. Radical cystectomy remains standard treatment for patients with muscle-invasive bladder cancer independent of age. Further studies to assess the differential effect of RC and the different types of urinary diversion on the health-related quality of life and metabolic consequences across age are necessary.

Author Contributions: Conceptualization, F.J. and M.R.; Data curation, M.R. and M.W.V.; Formal analysis, M.R. and H.Y.; Funding acquisition, M.R.; Investigation, F.J., H.Y. and M.R.; Methodology, M.R.; Project administration, A.S.; Resources, R.D.; Supervision, M.R. and M.F.; Validation, F.J., M.W.V. and O.E.; Visualization, A.S.; Writing—original draft, F.J., H.Y. and M.R.; Writing—review & editing, F.J., M.W.V., A.S., O.E., S.F.S., M.F. and M.R.

Acknowledgments: Hang Yu is supported by the China Scholarship Council.

Conflicts of Interest: Sharokh F. Shariat is consulting or advising the following: Astra Zeneca, BMS, Ferring, Ipsen, Jansen, MSD, Olympus, Pfizer, Pierre Fabre, Richard Wolf, Roche, Sanochemia, Urogen.

References

1. Siegel, R.L.; Miller, K.D.; Jemal, A. Cancer statistics, 2019. *CA Cancer J. Clin.* **2019**, *69*, 7–34. [CrossRef] [PubMed]
2. Guancial, E.A.; Roussel, B.; Bergsma, D.P.; Bylund, K.C.; Sahasrabudhe, D.; Messing, E.; Mohile, S.G.; Fung, C. Bladder cancer in the elderly patient: Challenges and solutions. *Clin. Interv. Aging* **2015**, *10*, 939–949. [CrossRef] [PubMed]
3. Shariat, S.F.; Milowsky, M.; Droller, M.J. Bladder cancer in the elderly. *Urol. Oncol.* **2009**, *27*, 653–667. [CrossRef] [PubMed]
4. Organization, W.H. *World Health Statistics 2018: Monitoring Health for the SDGs*; WHO: Geneva, Switzerland, 2018.
5. Abdollah, F.; Gandaglia, G.; Thuret, R.; Schmitges, J.; Tian, Z.; Jeldres, C.; Passoni, N.M.; Briganti, A.; Shariat, S.F.; Perrotte, P.; et al. Incidence, survival and mortality rates of stage-specific bladder cancer in United States: A trend analysis. *Cancer Epidemiol.* **2013**, *37*, 219–225. [CrossRef] [PubMed]
6. Leal, J.; Luengo-Fernandez, R.; Sullivan, R.; Witjes, J.A. Economic Burden of Bladder Cancer Across the European Union. *Eur. Urol.* **2016**, *69*, 438–447. [CrossRef] [PubMed]

7. Rink, M.; Crivelli, J.J.; Shariat, S.F.; Chun, F.K.; Messing, E.M.; Soloway, M.S. Smoking and Bladder Cancer: A Systematic Review of Risk and Outcomes. *Eur. Urol. Focus* **2015**, *1*, 17–27. [CrossRef]
8. Rink, M.; Furberg, H.; Zabor, E.C.; Xylinas, E.; Babjuk, M.; Pycha, A.; Lotan, Y.; Karakiewicz, P.I.; Novara, G.; Robinson, B.D.; et al. Impact of smoking and smoking cessation on oncologic outcomes in primary non-muscle-invasive bladder cancer. *Eur. Urol.* **2013**, *63*, 724–732. [CrossRef]
9. Rink, M.; Zabor, E.C.; Furberg, H.; Xylinas, E.; Ehdaie, B.; Novara, G.; Babjuk, M.; Pycha, A.; Lotan, Y.; Trinh, Q.D.; et al. Impact of smoking and smoking cessation on outcomes in bladder cancer patients treated with radical cystectomy. *Eur. Urol.* **2013**, *64*, 456–464. [CrossRef]
10. Denzinger, S.; Fritsche, H.M.; Otto, W.; Blana, A.; Wieland, W.F.; Burger, M. Early versus deferred cystectomy for initial high-risk pT1G3 urothelial carcinoma of the bladder: Do risk factors define feasibility of bladder-sparing approach? *Eur. Urol.* **2008**, *53*, 146–152. [CrossRef]
11. Lara, J.; Brunson, A.; Keegan, T.H.; Malogolowkin, M.; Pan, C.-X.; Yap, S.; deVere White, R. Determinants of survival for adolescents and young adults with urothelial bladder cancer: Results from the California Cancer Registry. *J. Urol.* **2016**, *196*, 1378–1382. [CrossRef]
12. Soave, A.; Dahlem, R.; Hansen, J.; Weisbach, L.; Minner, S.; Engel, O.; Kluth, L.A.; Chun, F.K.; Shariat, S.F.; Fisch, M.; et al. Gender-specific outcomes of bladder cancer patients: A stage-specific analysis in a contemporary, homogenous radical cystectomy cohort. *Eur. J. Surg. Oncol.* **2015**, *41*, 368–377. [CrossRef] [PubMed]
13. Soave, A.; Schmidt, S.; Dahlem, R.; Minner, S.; Engel, O.; Kluth, L.A.; John, L.M.; Hansen, J.; Schmid, M.; Sauter, G.; et al. Does the extent of variant histology affect oncological outcomes in patients with urothelial carcinoma of the bladder treated with radical cystectomy? *Urol. Oncol.* **2015**, *33*, 21.e21–21.e29. [CrossRef] [PubMed]
14. Rink, M.; Fajkovic, H.; Cha, E.K.; Gupta, A.; Karakiewicz, P.I.; Chun, F.K.; Lotan, Y.; Shariat, S.F. Death certificates are valid for the determination of cause of death in patients with upper and lower tract urothelial carcinoma. *Eur. Urol.* **2012**, *61*, 854–855. [CrossRef] [PubMed]
15. Institute, N.C. *Closing the Gap: Research and Care Imperatives for Adolescents and Young Adults with Cancer*; Institute, N.C.: Bethesda, MD, USA, 2006.
16. Feng, H.; Zhang, W.; Li, J.; Lu, X. Different patterns in the prognostic value of age for bladder cancer-specific survival depending on tumor stages. *Am. J. Cancer Res.* **2015**, *5*, 2090. [PubMed]
17. Nayak, J.G.; Gore, J.L.; Holt, S.K.; Wright, J.L.; Mossanen, M.; Dash, A. Patient-centered risk stratification of disposition outcomes following radical cystectomy. *Urol. Oncol. Semin. Orig. Investig.* **2016**, *34*, 235.e217–235.e223. [CrossRef] [PubMed]
18. Isbarn, H.; Jeldres, C.; Zini, L.; Perrotte, P.; Baillargeon-Gagne, S.; Capitanio, U.; Shariat, S.F.; Arjane, P.; Saad, F.; McCormack, M.; et al. A population based assessment of perioperative mortality after cystectomy for bladder cancer. *J. Urol.* **2009**, *182*, 70–77. [CrossRef] [PubMed]
19. Chromecki, T.F.; Mauermann, J.; Cha, E.K.; Svatek, R.S.; Fajkovic, H.; Karakiewicz, P.I.; Lotan, Y.; Tilki, D.; Bastian, P.J.; Volkmer, B.G.; et al. Multicenter validation of the prognostic value of patient age in patients treated with radical cystectomy. *World J. Urol.* **2012**, *30*, 753–759. [CrossRef] [PubMed]
20. Shariat, S.F.; Sfakianos, J.P.; Droller, M.J.; Karakiewicz, P.I.; Meryn, S.; Bochner, B.H. The effect of age and gender on bladder cancer: A critical review of the literature. *BJU Int.* **2010**, *105*, 300–308. [CrossRef] [PubMed]
21. Noon, A.P.; Martinsen, J.I.; Catto, J.W.F.; Pukkala, E. Occupation and Bladder Cancer Phenotype: Identification of Workplace Patterns That Increase the Risk of Advanced Disease Beyond Overall Incidence. *Eur. Urol. Focus* **2018**, *4*, 725–730. [CrossRef] [PubMed]
22. Crivelli, J.J.; Xylinas, E.; Kluth, L.A.; Rieken, M.; Rink, M.; Shariat, S.F. Effect of smoking on outcomes of urothelial carcinoma: A systematic review of the literature. *Eur. Urol.* **2014**, *65*, 742–754. [CrossRef]
23. Mathieu, R.; Lucca, I.; Klatte, T.; Babjuk, M.; Shariat, S.F. Trimodal therapy for invasive bladder cancer: Is it really equal to radical cystectomy? *Curr. Opin. Urol.* **2015**, *25*, 476–482. [CrossRef] [PubMed]
24. Ploussard, G.; Daneshmand, S.; Efstathiou, J.A.; Herr, H.W.; James, N.D.; Rodel, C.M.; Shariat, S.F.; Shipley, W.U.; Sternberg, C.N.; Thalmann, G.N.; et al. Critical Analysis of Bladder Sparing with Trimodal Therapy in Muscle-invasive Bladder Cancer: A Systematic Review. *Eur. Urol.* **2014**, *66*, 120–137. [CrossRef] [PubMed]

25. Knoedler, J.; Frank, I. Organ-sparing surgery in urology: Partial cystectomy. *Curr. Opin. Urol.* **2015**, *25*, 111–115. [CrossRef] [PubMed]
26. Katafigiotis, I.; Sfoungaristos, S.; Martini, A.; Stravodimos, K.; Anastasiou, I.; Mykoniatis, I.; Duvdevani, M.; Constantinides, C. Bladder Cancer to Patients Younger than 30 Years: A Retrospective Study and Review of the Literature. *Urol. J.* **2017**, *84*, 231–235. [CrossRef] [PubMed]
27. Telli, O.; Sarici, H.; Ozgur, B.C.; Doluoglu, O.G.; Sunay, M.M.; Bozkurt, S.; Eroglu, M. Urothelial cancer of bladder in young versus older adults: Clinical and pathological characteristics and outcomes. *Kaohsiung J. Med. Sci.* **2014**, *30*, 466–470. [CrossRef] [PubMed]
28. Yossepowitch, O.; Dalbagni, G. Transitional cell carcinoma of the bladder in young adults: Presentation, natural history and outcome. *J. Urol.* **2002**, *168*, 61–66. [CrossRef]
29. Lee, R.K.; Abol-Enein, H.; Artibani, W.; Bochner, B.; Dalbagni, G.; Daneshmand, S.; Fradet, Y.; Hautmann, R.E.; Lee, C.T.; Lerner, S.P.; et al. Urinary diversion after radical cystectomy for bladder cancer: Options, patient selection, and outcomes. *BJU Int.* **2014**, *113*, 11–23. [CrossRef] [PubMed]
30. Sung, J.M.; Martin, J.W.; Jefferson, F.A.; Sidhom, D.A.; Piranviseh, K.; Huang, M.; Nguyen, N.; Chang, J.; Ziogas, A.; Anton-Culver, H.; et al. Racial and Socioeconomic Disparities in Bladder Cancer Survival: Analysis of the California Cancer Registry. *Clin. Genitourin. Cancer* **2019**. [CrossRef]
31. Gild, P.; Wankowicz, S.A.; Sood, A.; von Landenberg, N.; Friedlander, D.F.; Alanee, S.; Chun, F.K.H.; Fisch, M.; Menon, M.; Trinh, Q.D.; et al. Racial disparity in quality of care and overall survival among black vs. white patients with muscle-invasive bladder cancer treated with radical cystectomy: A national cancer database analysis. *Urol. Oncol.* **2018**, *36*, 469.e1–469.e11. [CrossRef]
32. Dobruch, J.; Daneshmand, S.; Fisch, M.; Lotan, Y.; Noon, A.P.; Resnick, M.J.; Shariat, S.F.; Zlotta, A.R.; Boorjian, S.A. Gender and Bladder Cancer: A Collaborative Review of Etiology, Biology, and Outcomes. *Eur. Urol.* **2016**, *69*, 300–310. [CrossRef]
33. Svatek, R.S.; Shariat, S.F.; Lasky, R.E.; Skinner, E.C.; Novara, G.; Lerner, S.P.; Fradet, Y.; Bastian, P.J.; Kassouf, W.; Karakiewicz, P.I.; et al. The effectiveness of off-protocol adjuvant chemotherapy for patients with urothelial carcinoma of the urinary bladder. *Clin. Cancer Res.* **2010**, *16*, 4461–4467. [CrossRef] [PubMed]
34. Goossens-Laan, C.A.; Leliveld, A.M.; Verhoeven, R.H.; Kil, P.J.; de Bock, G.H.; Hulshof, M.C.; de Jong, I.J.; Coebergh, J.W. Effects of age and comorbidity on treatment and survival of patients with muscle-invasive bladder cancer. *Int. J. Cancer* **2014**, *135*, 905–912. [CrossRef] [PubMed]
35. Megwalu, I.I.; Vlahiotis, A.; Radwan, M.; Piccirillo, J.F.; Kibel, A.S. Prognostic impact of comorbidity in patients with bladder cancer. *Eur. Urol.* **2008**, *53*, 581–589. [CrossRef] [PubMed]
36. Fairey, A.S.; Jacobsen, N.E.; Chetner, M.P.; Mador, D.R.; Metcalfe, J.B.; Moore, R.B.; Rourke, K.F.; Todd, G.T.; Venner, P.M.; Voaklander, D.C.; et al. Associations between comorbidity, and overall survival and bladder cancer specific survival after radical cystectomy: Results from the Alberta Urology Institute Radical Cystectomy database. *J. Urol.* **2009**, *182*, 85–92. [CrossRef] [PubMed]

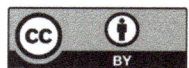

© 2019 by the authors. Licensee MDPI, Basel, Switzerland. This article is an open access article distributed under the terms and conditions of the Creative Commons Attribution (CC BY) license (http://creativecommons.org/licenses/by/4.0/).

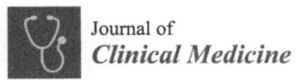

Article

Open Versus Robotic Cystectomy: A Propensity Score Matched Analysis Comparing Survival Outcomes

Marco Moschini [1,2,3], Stefania Zamboni [3], Francesco Soria [1,4], Romain Mathieu [1,5], Evanguelos Xylinas [6], Wei Shen Tan [7,8], John D Kelly [7,8], Giuseppe Simone [9], Anoop Meraney [10], Suprita Krishna [11], Badrinath Konety [11], Agostino Mattei [3], Philipp Baumeister [3], Livio Mordasini [3], Francesco Montorsi [2], Alberto Briganti [2], Andrea Gallina [2], Armando Stabile [2], Rafael Sanchez-Salas [12], Xavier Cathelineau [12], Michael Rink [13], Andrea Necchi [14], Pierre I. Karakiewicz [15], Morgan Rouprêt [16], Anthony Koupparis [17], Wassim Kassouf [18], Douglas S Scherr [19], Guillaume Ploussard [20], Stephen A. Boorjian [21], Yair Lotan [22], Prasanna Sooriakumaran [8,23] and Shahrokh F. Shariat [1,24,25,*]

1. Department of Urology, Comprehensive Cancer Center, Medical University of Vienna, Vienna General Hospital, A-1090 Vienna, Austria
2. Department of Urology, Urological Research Institute, San Raffaele Scientific Institute, 20132 Milan, Italy
3. Department of Urology, Luzerner Kantonsspital, Spitalstrasse, 6000 Luzern, Switzerland
4. Division of Urology, Department of Surgical Sciences, University of Studies of Torino, 10124 Turin, Italy
5. Department of Urology, Rennes University Hospital, 35000 Rennes, France
6. Department of Urology Bichat Hospital, Paris Descartes University, 75877 Paris, France
7. Division of Surgery and Intervention Science, University College London, London WC1E 6BT, UK
8. Department of Uro-Oncology, University College London Hospital NHS Foundation Trust, London W1T 4EU, UK
9. Department of Urology, "Regina Elena" National Cancer Institute, 00128 Rome, Italy
10. Urology Division, Hartford Healthcare Medical Group, Hartford, CT 06106, USA
11. Department of Urology, University of Minnesota, Minneapolis, MN 55455, USA
12. Department of Urology, L'Institut Mutualiste Montsouris, Université Paris Descartes, 75014 Paris, France
13. Department of Urology, University Medical Center Hamburg-Eppendorf, 20251 Hamburg, Germany
14. Fondazione IRCCS Istituto Nazionale dei Tumori, 20133 Milan, Italy
15. Cancer Prognostics and Health Outcomes Unit, University of Montreal Health Centre, Montreal, QC H4A 3J1, Canada
16. Sorbonne Université, GRC n°5, ONCOTYPE-URO, AP-HP, Hôpital Pitié-Salpêtrière, F-75013 Paris, France
17. Bristol Urological Institute, North Bristol NHS Trust, Southmead Hospital, Bristol BS10 5NB, UK
18. Department of Urology, McGill University Health Center, Montreal, QC H4A3J1, Canada
19. Department of Urology, Weill Cornell Medical College, New York-Presbyterian Hospital, New York, NY 10038, USA
20. Department of Urology, La Croix du sud Hospital, 314000 Toulouse, France
21. Department of Urology, Mayo Clinic, 200 First Street Southwest, Rochester, MN 55905, USA
22. Department of Urology, University of Texas Southwestern Medical Center, Dallas, TX 75390, USA
23. Department of Molecular Medicine and Surgery, Karolinska Institutet, 17177 Stockholm, Sweden
24. Department of Urology, Weill Cornell Medical College, New York Presbyterian Hospital, New York, NY 10021, USA
25. Department of Urology, The University of Texas M.D. Anderson Cancer Center, Houston, TX 77030, USA
* Correspondence: shahrokh.shariat@meduniwien.ac.at; Tel.: +1-40400-2615; Fax: +1-40400-2332

Received: 14 June 2019; Accepted: 6 August 2019; Published: 9 August 2019

Abstract: Background: To assess the differential effect of robotic assisted radical cystectomy (RARC) versus open radical cystectomy (ORC) on survival outcomes in matched analyses performed on a large multicentric cohort. Methods: The study included 9757 patients with urothelial bladder cancer (BCa) treated in a consecutive manner at each of 25 institutions. All patients underwent radical cystectomy with bilateral pelvic lymphadenectomy. To adjust for potential selection bias, propensity score matching 2:1 was performed with two ORC patients matched to one RARC patient.

The propensity-matched cohort included 1374 patients. Multivariable competing risk analyses accounting for death of other causes, tested association of surgical technique with recurrence and cancer specific mortality (CSM), before and after propensity score matching. Results: Overall, 767 (7.8%) patients underwent RARC and 8990 (92.2%) ORC. The median follow-up before and after propensity matching was 81 and 102 months, respectively. In the overall population, the 3-year recurrence rates and CSM were 37% vs. 26% and 34% vs. 24% for ORC vs. RARC (all p values > 0.1), respectively. On multivariable Cox regression analyses, RARC and ORC had similar recurrence and CSM rates before and after matching (all p values > 0.1). Conclusions: Patients treated with RARC and ORC have similar survival outcomes. This data is helpful in consulting patients until long term survival outcomes of level one evidence is available.

Keywords: bladder cancer; robotic-assisted; open; radical cystectomy; survival; propensity score

1. Introduction

Bladder cancer (BCa) is the second most common genitourinary malignancy with 81,190 estimated new diagnoses for 2018 in the United States alone [1]. Radical cystectomy (RC) with bilateral pelvic lymph node dissection (PLND) is the standard treatment for muscle invasive and very high risk non-muscle invasive BCa [2]. However, this procedure is associated with significant perioperative mortality and morbidity as a direct consequence of the complexity of the procedure and the characteristics of the population which is generally older and suffering from multiple comorbidities when compared to other surgical patients [3]. Minimally invasive surgeries, such as robotic assisted radical cystectomy (RARC), have been designed to improve surgical morbidity. Indeed, robotic-assisted radical surgery in urology has been shown to be associated with decreased blood loss, need for transfusion, and length of stay compared to open RC (ORC) in most studies [4–10].

While these perioperative benefits are generally accepted, the differential impact of RARC compared to ORC on survival outcomes remains debated with widely diverging opinions [4,11,12]. The RAZOR trial [13], a randomized, open-label, non-inferiority, phase 3 trial comparing ORC and RARC, found that RARC was non-inferior to open cystectomy for 2-year progression-free survival but did not report overall survival.

Given the shortage of prospective randomized trials comparing RARC to ORC, controlled data regarding the oncological risks and benefits are needed from well-designed retrospective multicenter studies.

Therefore, to address this unmet need, we collected complete data from BCa patients treated at academic centers to determine the impact of on survival outcomes of RARC compared to the standard ORC. We performed a propensity-matched analysis to limit the impact of selection bias on survival outcomes.

2. Experimental Section

2.1. Patients and Methods

We collected the data from 9757 patients treated with RC for non-metastatic UCB at 25 institutions. Patients were staged preoperatively with cross sectional imaging (mostly computerized tomography), bone scan when indicated and chest X-ray. Surgical specimens were processed according to standard pathologic procedures at each institution. Tumors were staged according to the 2009 American Joint Committee on Cancer-Union Internationale Centre le Cancer (AJCC/UICC) TNM classification. Tumor grade was assigned according to the 2003 WHO/International Society of Urologic Pathology (ISUP) consensus classification. STSM was defined as the presence of tumor at inked areas of soft tissue on the RC specimen [14,15]. Urethral and ureteral margins were not considered as STSM.

Lymphovascular invasion (LVI) was defined as the presence of tumor cells within an endothelium-lined space without underlying muscular walls [16,17].

2.2. Primary and Secondary End Points

The primary end-point was to compare survival outcomes of RARC with ORC. The secondary end-point was to evaluate survival outcomes of BCa patients treated with RARC. Overall recurrence and cancer-specific mortality (CSM) were defined as disease recurrence and death from disease, respectively.

2.3. Statistical Analyses

Descriptive statistics of categorical variables focused on frequencies and proportions. Means, medians, and interquartile ranges (IQR) were reported for continuously coded variables. The Mann–Whitney and chi-square tests were used to compare the statistical significance of differences in medians and proportions, respectively. Fine and Gray multivariable competing risk analyses tested the impact surgical technique and survival outcomes. Owing to inherent differences between patients undergoing ORC and RARC in terms of baseline patient and disease characteristics, we used a 2:1 propensity score matched analysis to adjust for the effects of these differences. The use of the propensity score method reduces the customary bias associated with the conventional multivariable modeling approach. The variables adjusted for were administration of neoadjuvant chemotherapy (NAC), grade, pathological T stage, lymph node status and age at surgery Subgroup analyses were performed. Statistical significance was considered at $p < 0.05$. Statistical analyses were performed using SPSS v.22.0 (IBM Corp., Armonk, NY, USA) and STATA 14 (Stata Corp., College Station, TX, USA).

3. Results

3.1. Clinicopathologic Characteristics (Entire Cohort)

Demographics and pathologic characteristics of the cohort stratified by surgical approach are shown in Table 1. Overall, 767 (7.8%) patients were treated with RARC and 8990 (92.2%) with ORC and most of the patients were men ($n = 7775$, 80%); median age was: 68 years (IQR: 60–74). About half of the patients ($n = 4248$, 45%) harbored pathological stage T3-T4, 6.7% had positive STSM ($n = 639$) and 24% ($n = 2276$) had lymph node metastases. There were no differences in age at surgery and gender between RARC and ORC patients (all p values > 0.1). Conversely, patients treated with RARC were more likely treated with NAC (26% vs. 3.6%) compared to patients treated with ORC and had less advanced diseases (pT3-pT4 stage: 40% vs. 46% and lymph node metastasis 22% vs. 24%). RARC patients were less likely to receive adjuvant chemotherapy compared to ORC patients (13% vs. 21%).

Table 1. Clinicopathologic demographics of 9757 patients with bladder cancer treated with radical cystectomy according type of surgery.

Variables	Overall ($n = 9757$, 100%)	RARC ($n = 767$, 7.8%)	ORC ($n = 8990$, 92%)	p Value
Age, years Mean Median (IQR)	67 68 (60–74)	67 68 (62–74)	67 68 (60–74)	0.2
Gender Male Female	7775 (79%) 1981 (20%)	612 (80%) 115 (20%)	7163 (80%) 1827 (20%)	0.9
Neoadjuvant chemotherapy	520 (5.3%)	198 (26%)	322 (3.6%)	<0.001

Table 1. Cont.

Variables	Overall (n = 9757, 100%)	RARC (n = 767, 7.8%)	ORC (n = 8990, 92%)	p Value
Pathological T stage				
pT0-pT1	2908 (31%)	368 (48%)	2540 (29%)	
pT2	2239 (24%)	93 (12%)	2146 (25%)	<0.001
pT3-pT4	4248 (45%)	305 (40%)	3943 (46%)	
High grade	8734 (94%)	361 (76%)	8373 (94%)	<0.001
LNI	2276 (24%)	158 (22%)	2118 (24%)	0.001
Nodes removed, number				
Mean	20	21	20	0.001
Median (IQR)	16 (10–26)	20 (13–28)	16 (9–25)	
Positive surgical margins	639 (6.7%)	107 (10.0%)	532 (6.3%)	<0.001
LVI	3007 (33%)	25 (27%)	2982 (34%)	0.2
Adjuvant chemotherapy	1828 (19%)	85 (13%)	1743 (20.9%)	<0.001

RARC: robotic assisted radical cystectomy, ORC: open radical cystectomy, IQR: interquartile range, LNI: lymph node invasion, LVI: lymphovascular invasion.

3.2. Clinicopathologic Characteristics (Adjusted Cohort)

Demographics and pathologic characteristics of the cohort after propensity matching, stratified by surgical approach are reported in Table 2. After the propensity matching, 420 (33%) patients were treated with RARC and 840 (67%) with ORC; no differences were recorded between ORC and RARC patients considering age, gender, NAC usage, pathological T stage, pathologic grade, and lymph node invasion (all $p > 0.1$). On the other hand, patients treated with RARC recorded higher rate of positive STSM compared to ORC group (11% vs. 6.3%).

Table 2. Clinicopathologic characteristics of 1374 patients with bladder cancer treated with radical cystectomy, comparing robot assisted radical cystectomy (RARC) and open radical cystectomy (ORC) cohorts after propensity matching.

Variables	Overall (n = 1374, 100%)	RARC (n = 420, 33%)	ORC (n = 840, 67%)	p Value
Age, years				
Mean	66	66	66	0.9
Median (IQR)	67 (59–73)	67 (61–72)	67 (51–72)	
Gender				
Male	1003 (80%)	365 (80%)	728 (79%)	0.9
Female	257 (20%)	93 (20%)	188 (21%)	
Neoadjuvant chemotherapy	456 (33%)	1162 (35%)	294 (32%)	0.2
Pathological T stage				
pT0-pT1	535 (39%)	189 (41%)	346 (38%)	
pT2	208 (15%)	52 (11%)	156 (17%)	0.4
pT3-pT4	631 (46%)	217 (47%)	414 (52%)	
High grade	1075 (78%)	348 (76%)	727 (79%)	0.1
Nodes removed, number				
Mean	19	22	17	0.001
Median (IQR)	16 (10–25)	19 (14–28)	14 (8–24)	

Table 2. Cont.

Variables	Overall (n = 1374, 100%)	RARC (n = 420, 33%)	ORC (n = 840, 67%)	p Value
LNI	318 (23%)	109 (24%)	209 (23%)	0.6
Positive surgical margins	115 (8.4%)	52 (11%)	63 (7.0%)	0.006
LVI	302 (32%)	23 (45%)	282 (32%)	0.04
Adjuvant chemotherapy	211 (16%)	45 (12%)	166 (18%)	0.004

RARC: robotic assisted radical cystectomy, ORC: open radical cystectomy, IQR: interquartile range, LNI: lymph node invasion, LVI: lymphovascular invasion.

3.3. Survival Analyses in the Entire Cohort (Unadjusted Cohort)

The median follow-ups before and after propensity matching were 81 and 102 months, respectively. The 3-year recurrence rates, CSM and OM were 37% vs. 26%, 34% vs. 24% and 47% vs. 34% for ORC vs. RARC (Figure 1, all p values > 0.1), respectively. On multivariable Cox regression analyses adjusting for standard clinico-pathologic characteristics, no significant differences were found between RARC and ORC in overall recurrence and CSM (Table 3, $p > 0.1$).

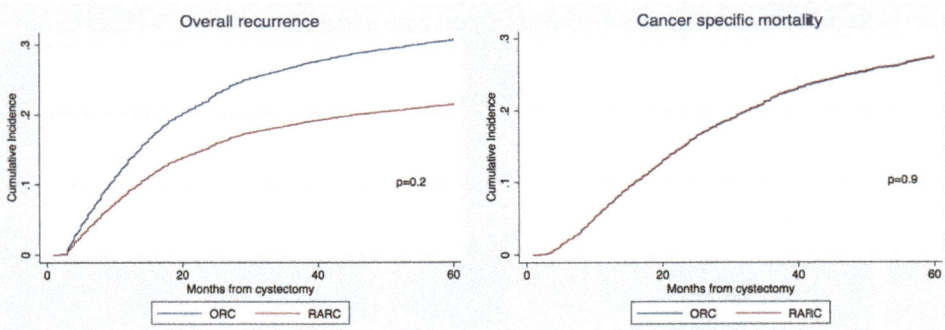

Figure 1. Cumulative incidence of recurrence and cancer specific mortality on overall population of patients with non-metastatic bladder cancer (BCa) treated with radical cystectomy according the type of surgery (ORC vs. RARC).

Table 3. Multivariable competing risk analyses predicting the risk of overall recurrence and cancer specific mortality (CSM) in patients treated with radical cystectomy in overall patients.

Variables	Overall Recurrence		CSM	
	HR (CI 95%)	p Value	HR (CI 95%)	p Value
Gender (male vs. female)	1.07 (0.97–1.17)	0.1	1.15 (1.04–1.27)	0.005
Age, years	1.00 (0.99–1.00)	0.5	1.00 (0.99–1.00)	0.052
RARC approach	0.65 (0.34–1.26)	0.2	1.00 (0.45–2.24)	0.9
pT stage				
pT0-pT1	Ref	Ref	Ref	Ref
pT2	1.35 (1.18–1.55)	<0.001	1.49 (1.27–1.73)	<0.001
pT3-4	2.10 (1.84–2.40)	<0.001	2.62 (2.27–3.03)	<0.001
pN+	1.68 (1.51–1.86)	<0.001	2.09 (1.88–2.33)	<0.001
Nodes removed	0.99 (0.99–1.00)	0.3	0.99 (0.99–1.00)	0.04
High grade vs. low	2.53 (1.73–3.71)	<0.001	2.37 (1.56–3.60)	<0.001

Table 3. *Cont.*

Variables	Overall Recurrence		CSM	
	HR (CI 95%)	*p* Value	HR (CI 95%)	*p* Value
LVI	1.44 (1.31–1.57)	<0.001	1.33 (1.21–1.46)	<0.001
Positive surgical margins	1.43 (1.25–1.65)	<0.001	1.64 (1.42–1.90)	<0.001
Neoadjuvant chemotherapy	1.69 (1.36–2.10)	<0.001	1.45 (1.15–1.85)	0.002
Adjuvant chemotherapy	1.18 (1.06–1.31)	0.001	0.89 (0.80–0.99)	0.03

CSM: cancer specific mortality, HR: Hazard ratio, CI: confidence interval, RARC: robotic assisted radical cystectomy, LVI: lymphovascular invasion.

3.4. Survival Analyses after Propensity Matching (Adjusted Cohort)

The 3-year recurrence and CSM were 31% vs. 29% and 27% vs. 26% for ORC vs. RARC, respectively (Figure 2, all *p* values > 0.3), respectively. On multivariable Cox regression analyses adjusting for standard clinicopathologic characteristics, RARC was again associated with similar overall recurrence and CSM compared to ORC (Table 4, *p* > 0.3).

Table 4. Multivariable competing risk analyses predicting the risk of overall recurrence and CSM in patients treated with radical cystectomy after propensity matching.

Variables	Overall Recurrence		CSM	
	HR (CI 95%)	*p* Value	HR (CI 95%)	*p* Value
Gender (male vs. female)	1.09 (0.80–1.48)	0.6	1.23 (0.91–1.67)	0.1
Age, years	1.00 (0.99–1.01)	0.5	1.01 (0.99–1.02)	0.09
RARC approach	0.76 (0.39–1.47)	0.4	1.34 (0.49–2.36)	0.8
pT stage				
pT0-1	Ref	Ref	Ref	Ref
pT2	1.21 (0.77–1.90)	0.3	1.34 (0.84–2.15)	0.2
pT3-4	1.57 (1.04–2.37)	0.03	2.17 (1.40–3.35)	<0.001
pN+	1.43 (1.05–1.94)	0.02	2.33 (1.71–3.16)	<0.001
Nodes removed	0.99 (0.98–1.00)	0.3	0.98 (0.97–0.99)	0.01
High grade vs. low	3.20 (1.55–6.59)	0.002	3.60 (1.62–7.98)	0.002
LVI	1.85 (1.37–2.49)	<0.001	1.27 (0.96–1.70)	0.09
Positive surgical margins	1.12 (0.74–1.69)	0.5	1.30 (0.84–2.01)	0.2
Neoadjuvant chemotherapy	1.96 (1.51–2.54)	<0.001	1.34 (1.02–1.76)	0.03
Adjuvant chemotherapy	1.29 (0.94–1.77)	0.1	0.77 (0.56–1.06)	0.1

CSM: cancer specific mortality, HR: Hazard ratio, CI: confidence interval, RARC: robotic assisted radical cystectomy, LVI: lymphovascular invasion.

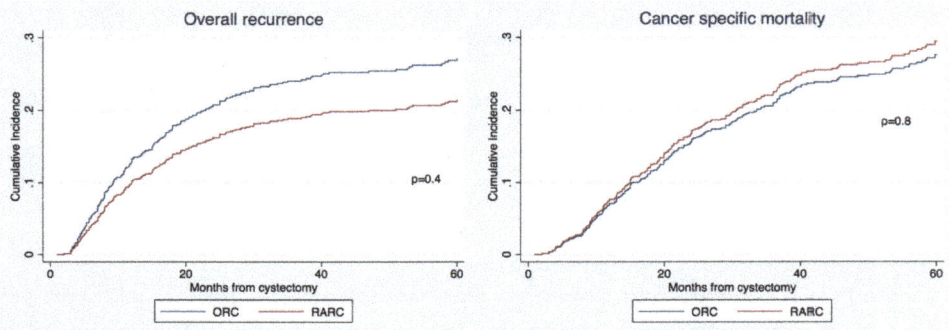

Figure 2. Cumulative incidence of recurrence and cancer specific mortality of patients with non-metastatic BCa treated with radical cystectomy according the type of surgery (ORC vs. RARC) after 2:1 propensity matching for age, pathological T stage, pathological N stage, neoadjuvant chemotherapy (NAC) and grade.

4. Discussion

The adoption of RARC is growing rapidly, but the majority of radical cystectomies continues to be performed by a conventional open approach. The majority of the current data from RARC series which tested perioperative and short term oncological outcomes did not test equivalence regarding long term survival outcomes [18–21]. Several retrospective series raised, indeed, some concerns regarding the oncological safety of the robotic approach [22]. On the other hand, two different prospective trials found no differences in survival outcomes between the two surgical approaches [13,23].

In this multicenter study, we evaluated the survival outcomes of the largest international cohort of bladder cancer patients treated with either ORC or RARC. Patients were treated in both European and American referral centers, collecting data from almost 1000 RARC and matching them with almost 9000 ORC patients. This manuscript follows two previous publications [10,21] from the same collaboration, evaluating for the first time the impact of survival and on peri-operative outcomes demonstrating an advantage of RARC in blood loss and length of stay. New centers were added to this manuscript in respect of the previous publications and the match of the final database was performed separately for each study on the bases of the main aim of each project.

We found that RARC and ORC share similar survival outcomes, both on univariable and multivariable analyses controlled for established prognostic factors. We performed propensity matching to minimize the risk of selection bias adjusting for pathological stage, lymph node status, and age at surgery. Even in this setting we confirmed that the RARC approach is associated with similar recurrence and CSM rates compared to ORC. These results were obtained with a median follow-up before and after propensity matching of 81 and 102 months, respectively. Similarly to our previous manuscript [21], we found a positive surgical margin status higher than 10% in patients treated with RARC. However, this was consistently higher than in patients treated with RARC compared to patients treated with ORC. Despite these differences, this had no impact on survival outcomes when adjusted for all the available confounders in the multivariable model.

Our results confirm the findings of the RAZOR trial [13], an open label, randomized, phase 3, non-inferiority trial comparing RARC versus ORC. A total of 152 patients were included in the ORC group and compared to 150 patients treated with RARC, reporting similar 2-year progression free survival rates. Bochner et al. [23], in a prospective, randomized trial compared 60 and 58 patients treated with RARC and ORC, respectively. No differences were found considering recurrence, cancer survival, or overall survival. Previously, Bochner et al. [18] reported in a single center prospective randomized trial, an advantage in terms of mean intraoperative blood loss for the RARC group but longer operative times compared to ORC. However, no survival outcomes were reported. Similarly, in the prospective trial of Khan et al. [24] and Nix et al. [20] survival outcomes were not analyzed. Given the paucity of prospective data analyzing survival outcomes of RARC patients, new long term level one evidence are required.

Several retrospective series focused on mid-long-term survival outcomes [22,25]. Nguyen at al. [22] analyzed 383 consecutive patients treated with ORC (120) or RARC (263) between 2001 and 2014 at a single institution. With a median follow up of 30 months (for ORC) and 23 months (for RARC), they reported similar recurrence rates with an increasing risk of experiencing extrapelvic lymph node recurrence and peritoneal carcinomatoses for RARC patients. Our analyses did not include the type of recurrence limiting our ability to test this aspect; but we found a similar overall recurrence risk for patients treated with RARC when compared to ORC.

Hu et al. [25], using the SEER database compared 439 patients treated with RARC and 7308 treated with ORC. These authors observed an increasing trend in RARC utilization over the study period and with a median follow up of 44 months, they found no survival differences between the two techniques. However, as recognized by the authors themselves, they analyzed only a small RARC cohort treated by many different centers in their learning in some cases. In a recent systematic review and meta-analyses [26], five studies with a total of 540 participants were included. Authors found no differences in disease progression and local recurrences between patients treated with RARC and ORC. Finally, a recent large retrospective study analyzed the outcomes of RARC versus ORC in the selected population of patients who had received perioperative chemotherapy (in the neoadjuvant or adjuvant setting). No difference was found in multivariable analyses in the rate of positive surgical margins, rate of neobladder diversion, recurrence, and overall survival [27].

Our study represents the largest multicenter collaboration analyzing survival outcomes of patients affected by bladder cancer analyzing the effect of the RARC approach. Our analyses differentiate itself from previous reports including referral centers but excluding low case volume and learning curves which may lead to suboptimal outcomes. Our study comprises the largest available cohort to date analyzing survival outcomes in RARC patients. Despite several strengths, our study is not devoid of limitations. First and foremost, we recognize that our study is limited by its observational nature, and thus our results should be interpreted within the limits of its retrospective design. Second, we did not perform a central review of all specimens and therefore relied on the dedication and attention of the local uro-pathologists. Third, we did not include data regarding urinary diversion that might have an influence on survival outcomes. On the other hand, previous literature failed to prove any differences regarding different urinary diversion in RARC patients supporting the hypothesis of similar survival outcomes between these two groups [28]. Patients treated in academic centers are more prone to be treated with RARC as compared to ORC [8], moreover, differences exist regarding tumor characteristics, patient characteristics, and year of surgery (with an increasing tendency to perform a RARC) [29,30]. These elements can only partially be adjusted for with a propensity match analysis; we are aware that our results need to be confirmed in a controlled randomized trial. In this regard, a high proportion of RARC patients were found with pT0 disease at RC specimen, that might indicate a selection bias that can be only partially mitigated by the propensity matching analyses.

5. Conclusions

Patients treated with RARC were found with an increased rate of positive surgical margin compared to those treated with ORC. However, no differences regarding overall recurrence rate and survival were found between the two study groups. These results were confirmed in propensity score matched analyses adjusted for all the major confounders. High quality prospective trials are warranted to support the long-term oncological safety of RARC.

Author Contributions: M.M.: conceptualization, methodology, validation, formal analysis, investigation, data curation, writing original draft preparation, writing—review and editing; S.Z.: conceptualization, methodology, validation, formal analysis, investigation, data curation, writing—review and editing; F.S., R.M., E.X., W.S.T., J.D.K., G.S., A.M. (Anoop Meraney), S.K., B.K., A.M. (Agostino Mattei), P.B., L.M., F.M., A.B., A.G., A.S., R.S.-S., X.C., M.R., A.N., P.I.K., M.R. A.K., W.K., D.S.S., G.P., S.A.B., Y.L., P.S.: methodology, validation, data curation, writing—review and editing; S.F.S.: conceptualization, methodology, validation, investigation, data curation, writing—review and editing, project administration.

Acknowledgments: On behalf of the European Association of Urology-Young Academic Urologists (EAU-YAU), Urothelial carcinoma working group.

Conflicts of Interest: The authors declare no conflict of interest.

References

1. Siegel, R.L.; Miller, K.D.; Jemal, A. Cancer statistics, 2018. *CA Cancer J. Clin.* **2018**, *68*, 7–30. [CrossRef] [PubMed]
2. Babjuk, M.; Böhle, A.; Burger, M.; Capoun, O.; Cohen, D.; Compérat, E.M.; Hernández, V.; Kaasinen, E.; Palou, J.; Rouprêt, M.; et al. EAU Guidelines on Non-Muscle-invasive Urothelial Carcinoma of the Bladder: Update 2016. *Eur. Urol.* **2016**, *71*, 447–461. [CrossRef] [PubMed]
3. Moschini, M.; Simone, G.; Stenzl, A.; Gill, I.S.; Catto, J. Critical Review of Outcomes from Radical Cystectomy: Can Complications from Radical Cystectomy Be Reduced by Surgical Volume and Robotic Surgery? *Eur. Urol. Focus* **2016**, *2*, 19–29. [CrossRef] [PubMed]
4. Challacombe, B.J.; Bochner, B.H.; Dasgupta, P.; Gill, I.; Guru, K.; Herr, H.; Mottrie, A.; Pruthi, R.; Redorta, J.P.; Wiklund, P. The Role of Laparoscopic and Robotic Cystectomy in the Management of Muscle-Invasive Bladder Cancer with Special Emphasis on Cancer Control and Complications. *Eur. Urol.* **2011**, *60*, 767–775. [CrossRef] [PubMed]
5. Yu, H.-Y.; Hevelone, N.D.; Lipsitz, S.R.; Kowalczyk, K.J.; Nguyen, P.L.; Choueiri, T.K.; Kibel, A.S.; Hu, J.C. Comparative Analysis of Outcomes and Costs Following Open Radical Cystectomy Versus Robot-Assisted Laparoscopic Radical Cystectomy: Results From the US Nationwide Inpatient Sample. *Eur. Urol.* **2012**, *61*, 1239–1244. [CrossRef] [PubMed]
6. Styn, N.R.; Montgomery, J.S.; Wood, D.P.; Hafez, K.S.; Lee, C.T.; Tallman, C.; He, C.; Crossley, H.; Hollenbeck, B.K.; Weizer, A.Z. Matched comparison of robotic-assisted and open radical cystectomy. *Urology* **2012**, *79*, 1303–1309. [CrossRef]
7. Ng, C.K.; Kauffman, E.C.; Lee, M.-M.; Otto, B.J.; Portnoff, A.; Ehrlich, J.R.; Schwartz, M.J.; Wang, G.J.; Scherr, D.S. A Comparison of Postoperative Complications in Open versus Robotic Cystectomy. *Eur. Urol.* **2010**, *57*, 274–282. [CrossRef]
8. Hanna, N.; Leow, J.J.; Sun, M.; Friedlander, D.F.; Seisen, T.; Abdollah, F.; Lipsitz, S.R.; Menon, M.; Kibel, A.S.; Bellmunt, J.; et al. Comparative effectiveness of robot-assisted vs. open radical cystectomy. *Urol. Oncol. Semin. Orig. Investig.* **2018**, *36*, 88.e1–88.e9. [CrossRef]
9. Hussein, A.A.; May, P.R.; Jing, Z.; Ahmed, Y.E.; Wijburg, C.J.; Canda, A.E.; Dasgupta, P.; Khan, M.S.; Menon, M.; Peabody, J.O.; et al. Outcomes of Intracorporeal Urinary Diversion after Robot-Assisted Radical Cystectomy: Results from the International Robotic Cystectomy Consortium. *J. Urol.* **2018**, *199*, 1302–1311. [CrossRef]
10. Soria, F.; Moschini, M.; D'Andrea, D.; Abufaraj, M.; Foerster, B.; Mathiéu, R.; Gust, K.M.; Gontero, P.; Simone, G.; Meraney, A.; et al. Comparative Effectiveness in Perioperative Outcomes of Robotic versus Open Radical Cystectomy: Results from a Multicenter Contemporary Retrospective Cohort Study. *Eur. Urol. Focus* **2018**. [CrossRef]
11. Martin, A.D.; Nunez, R.N.; Pacelli, A.; Woods, M.E.; Davis, R.; Thomas, R.; Andrews, P.E.; Castle, E.P. Robot-assisted radical cystectomy: Intermediate survival results at a mean follow-up of 25 months. *BJU Int.* **2010**, *105*, 1706–1709. [CrossRef]
12. Jonsson, M.N.; Adding, L.C.; Hosseini, A.; Schumacher, M.C.; Volz, D.; Nilsson, A.; Carlsson, S.; Wiklund, N.P. Robot-Assisted Radical Cystectomy with Intracorporeal Urinary Diversion in Patients with Transitional Cell Carcinoma of the Bladder. *Eur. Urol.* **2011**, *60*, 1066–1073. [CrossRef] [PubMed]

13. Parekh, D.J.; Reis, I.M.; Castle, E.P.; Gonzalgo, M.L.; Woods, M.E.; Svatek, R.S.; Weizer, A.Z.; Konety, B.R.; Tollefson, M.; Krupski, T.L.; et al. Robot-assisted radical cystectomy versus open radical cystectomy in patients with bladder cancer (RAZOR): An open-label, randomised, phase 3, non-inferiority trial. *Lancet* **2018**, *391*, 2525–2536. [CrossRef]
14. Novara, G.; Svatek, R.S.; Karakiewicz, P.I.; Skinner, E.; Ficarra, V.; Fradet, Y.; Lotan, Y.; Isbarn, H.; Capitanio, U.; Bastian, P.J.; et al. Soft Tissue Surgical Margin Status is a Powerful Predictor of Outcomes After Radical Cystectomy: A Multicenter Study of More Than 4400 Patients. *J. Urol.* **2010**, *183*, 2165–2170. [CrossRef] [PubMed]
15. Xylinas, E.; Rink, M.; Novara, G.; Green, D.A.; Clozel, T.; Fritsche, H.M.; Guillonneau, B.; Lotan, Y.; Kassouf, W.; Tilki, D.; et al. Predictors of survival in patients with soft tissue surgical margin involvement at radical cystectomy. *Ann. Surg. Oncol.* **2013**, *20*, 1027–1034. [CrossRef] [PubMed]
16. Mathieu, R.; Lucca, I.; Rouprêt, M.; Briganti, A.; Shariat, S.F. The prognostic role of lymphovascular invasion in urothelial carcinoma of the bladder. *Nat. Rev. Urol.* **2016**, *13*, 471–479. [CrossRef]
17. Shariat, S.F.; Khoddami, S.M.; Saboorian, H.; Koeneman, K.S.; Sagalowsky, A.I.; Cadeddu, J.A.; McConnell, J.D.; Holmes, M.N.; Roehrborn, C.G. Lymphovascular Invasion is a Pathological Feature of Biologically Aggressive Disease in Patients Treated with Radical Prostatectomy. *J. Urol.* **2004**, *171*, 1122–1127. [CrossRef]
18. Bochner, B.H.; Sjoberg, D.D.; Laudone, V.P. A Randomized Trial of Robot-Assisted Laparoscopic Radical Cystectomy. *N. Engl. J. Med.* **2014**, *371*, 389–390. [CrossRef]
19. Parekh, D.J.; Messer, J.; Fitzgerald, J.; Ercole, B.; Svatek, R. Perioperative outcomes and oncologic efficacy from a pilot prospective randomized clinical trial of open versus robotic assisted radical cystectomy. *J. Urol.* **2013**, *189*, 474–479. [CrossRef]
20. Nix, J.; Smith, A.; Kurpad, R.; Nielsen, M.E.; Wallen, E.M.; Pruthi, R.S. Prospective randomized controlled trial of robotic versus open radical cystectomy for bladder cancer: Perioperative and pathologic results. *Eur. Urol.* **2010**, *57*, 196–201. [CrossRef]
21. Moschini, M.; Soria, F.; Mathieu, R.; Xylinas, E.; D'Andrea, D.; Tan, W.S.; Kelly, J.D.; Simone, G.; Tuderti, G.; Meraney, A.; et al. Propensity-score-matched comparison of soft tissue surgical margins status between open and robotic-assisted radical cystectomy. *Urol. Oncol. Semin. Orig. Investig.* **2019**, *37*, 179.e1–179.e7. [CrossRef] [PubMed]
22. Nguyen, D.P.; Awamlh, B.A.H.A.; Wu, X.; O'Malley, P.; Inoyatov, I.M.; Ayangbesan, A.; Faltas, B.M.; Christos, P.J.; Scherr, D.S. Recurrence Patterns After Open and Robot-assisted Radical Cystectomy for Bladder Cancer. *Eur. Urol.* **2015**, *68*, 399–405. [CrossRef] [PubMed]
23. Bochner, B.H.; Dalbagni, G.; Marzouk, K.H.; Sjoberg, D.D.; Lee, J.; Donat, S.M.; Coleman, J.A.; Vickers, A.; Herr, H.W.; Laudone, V.P. Randomized Trial Comparing Open Radical Cystectomy and Robot-assisted Laparoscopic Radical Cystectomy: Oncologic Outcomes. *Eur. Urol.* **2018**, *74*, 465–471. [CrossRef] [PubMed]
24. Khan, M.S.; Gan, C.; Ahmed, K.; Ismail, A.F.; Watkins, J.; Summers, J.A.; Peacock, J.L.; Rimington, P.; Dasgupta, P. A Single-centre Early Phase Randomised Controlled Three-arm Trial of Open, Robotic, and Laparoscopic Radical Cystectomy (CORAL). *Eur. Urol.* **2016**, *69*, 613–621. [CrossRef] [PubMed]
25. Hu, J.C.; Chughtai, B.; O'Malley, P.; Halpern, J.A.; Mao, J.; Scherr, D.S.; Hershman, D.L.; Wright, J.D.; Sedrakyan, A. Perioperative Outcomes, Health Care Costs, and Survival After Robotic-assisted Versus Open Radical Cystectomy: A National Comparative Effectiveness Study. *Eur. Urol.* **2016**, *70*, 195–202. [CrossRef] [PubMed]
26. Sathianathen, N.J.; Kalapara, A.; Frydenberg, M.; Lawrentschuk, N.; Weight, C.J.; Parekh, D.; Konety, B.R. Robotic Assisted Radical Cystectomy vs Open Radical Cystectomy: Systematic Review and Meta-Analysis. *J. Urol.* **2018**. [CrossRef] [PubMed]
27. Necchi, A.; Pond, G.R.; Smaldone, M.C.; Pal, S.K.; Chan, K.; Wong, Y.-N.; Viterbo, R.; Sonpavde, G.; Harshman, L.C.; Crabb, S.; et al. Robot-assisted Versus Open Radical Cystectomy in Patients Receiving Perioperative Chemotherapy for Muscle-invasive Bladder Cancer: The Oncologist's Perspective from a Multicentre Study. *Eur. Urol. Focus* **2018**, *4*, 937–945. [CrossRef]
28. Pyun, J.H.; Kim, H.K.; Cho, S.; Kang, S.G.; Cheon, J.; Lee, J.G.; Kim, J.J.; Kang, S.H. Robot-Assisted Radical Cystectomy with Total Intracorporeal Urinary Diversion: Comparative Analysis with Extracorporeal Urinary Diversion. *J. Laparoendosc. Adv. Surg. Tech.* **2016**, *26*, 349–355. [CrossRef]

29. Leow, J.J.; Reese, S.W.; Jiang, W.; Lipsitz, S.R.; Bellmunt, J.; Trinh, Q.-D.; Chung, B.I.; Kibel, A.S.; Chang, S.L. Propensity-Matched Comparison of Morbidity and Costs of Open and Robot-Assisted Radical Cystectomies: A Contemporary Population-Based Analysis in the United States. *Eur. Urol.* **2014**, *66*, 569–576. [CrossRef]
30. Monn, M.F.; Cary, K.C.; Kaimakliotis, H.Z.; Flack, C.K.; Koch, M.O. National trends in the utilization of robotic-assisted radical cystectomy: An analysis using the Nationwide Inpatient Sample. *Urol. Oncol. Semin. Orig. Investig.* **2014**, *32*, 785–790. [CrossRef]

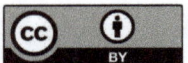

© 2019 by the authors. Licensee MDPI, Basel, Switzerland. This article is an open access article distributed under the terms and conditions of the Creative Commons Attribution (CC BY) license (http://creativecommons.org/licenses/by/4.0/).

MDPI
St. Alban-Anlage 66
4052 Basel
Switzerland
Tel. +41 61 683 77 34
Fax +41 61 302 89 18
www.mdpi.com

Journal of Clinical Medicine Editorial Office
E-mail: jcm@mdpi.com
www.mdpi.com/journal/jcm

www.ingramcontent.com/pod-product-compliance
Lightning Source LLC
LaVergne TN
LVHW070044120526
838202LV00101B/430